I0449880

AND THE TIGERS COME AGAIN

Basil Jay

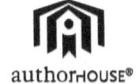

authorHOUSE®

AuthorHouse™ UK Ltd.
500 Avebury Boulevard
Central Milton Keynes, MK9 2BE
www.authorhouse.co.uk
Phone: 08001974150

© 2011 Basil Jay. All rights reserved.

No part of this book may be reproduced, stored in a retrieval system, or transmitted by any means without the written permission of the author.

First published by AuthorHouse 6/22/2011

ISBN: 978-1-4567-7555-1 (sc)

Any people depicted in stock imagery provided by Thinkstock are models, and such images are being used for illustrative purposes only. Certain stock imagery © Thinkstock.

This book is printed on acid-free paper.

Because of the dynamic nature of the Internet, any web addresses or links contained in this book may have changed since publication and may no longer be valid. The views expressed in this work are solely those of the author and do not necessarily reflect the views of the publisher, and the publisher hereby disclaims any responsibility for them.

I dedicate this book to
My Mother

But also to
Betty, Pippa, Diane
Pam, Celia and Heather

And all the Ladies who display real courage
In the face of adversity

COURAGE
From a poem by John Alfred Eades
Written sometime between Dunkirk 1940
And his death from his wounds in November 1944

Hope

Death holds no pain, no fears
As I look down my remaining years;
*I hold, so hard, that **will** to live*
That cherished hope that I can give
Those whom I love, a future bright,
For them, I pray, for them, I fight.

Death

On equal terms once more we'll meet
I will battle hard in your defeat,
Though hard, I know, sadly not long
The fight is on, will death begone
The victor, know I, will be thee,
But many fights, yet let there be

Release

My earthly life draws to its close
I leave, loved ones, and join those
Who free again, are in some unknown sphere,
Body cast, but soul immortal be
Friends gone before will look, will smile, will cheer
And I will be, at last oh Lord, with thee

CONTENTS

PROLOGUE –

MAY 2007

"Well, well, well" she said with a resigned look, "Basil, what brings you here today?" I beamed her a smile that sent a warm tingle racing up her spine.

"I suppose you could say, a clot" I answered

"A clot" she repeated,

"A clot" I agreed, "and a little finger"

"A little finger" *in a raised eyebrows sort of a voice*

"And a thumb" I said with a grimace

"And a thumb". She repeated, both the words and the grimace.

"And a badly sunburned lip" I said, pouting to show her a badly sunburned lip.

"Anything else?" she said

"Only my hernia" I added with a smile

"You are an enigma" she said in an *'of all the clinics, in all the world'* sort of a voice. "You better start from the top.

"Well", I began, making myself comfortable for one of my favourite audiences, "I suppose *the top* was the top of an escalator in Gatwick Airport" I paused, "or perhaps, more accurately, *the top,* was the *bottom* of the escalator, because that is where I think my current troubles began"

"Basil" she interrupted. "It's the end of a busy day, this is a doctor's surgery, you are the last of my long list of patients, and I want to go home and have a hot bath and a glass of wine", I could sense that the warm tingle was beginning to cool, "please be brief".

"I had just spent a few days in Bulgaria, on my own" I continued, unabashed.

"Basil!", Ice was beginning to form, the warm glow had now all but gone.

"Well I wasn't exactly on my own", I felt I had to explain. "I was with Sharron", I felt a need to explain further since misunderstandings in a small village can have catastrophic effects. "Sharron is the CEO of my old company; we were in Bulgaria to......"

Basil. *Now a hint of steel in her voice.* I took the hint.

"I caught the plane from Sofia airport" I paused to explain "that's the capital of Bulgaria your know"

"No" she said wearily, "I did not know that Bulgaria had an airport as its capital" I gave her a well deserved smile for demonstrating that she had not quite, yet, lost the will to live. Then I continued

"at 3 o'clock in the morning and I fell down the escalator at Gatwick at 2.30 the next afternoon" I finished lamely.

"You hurt your leg" she said

"No" I replied, I cut my head, damaged my hand, and ruined my shirt.

"But you just said you finished lamely" she said. No she didn't, I just made that up.

"You better start at the beginning then" she continued, suddenly forgetting the hot bath, the glass of wine and the desire to go home. I could almost see the steam rising from her spine as the warm glow returned. I was relieved; I just hate it when common sense gets in the way of a good story.

"The plane from Sofia arrived in Gatwick at 9.am UK time, I had hand luggage only, so was in transfer departures by 9.30 knowing that the plane did not take off for Tenerife until three in the afternoon"

"A long wait she said" suddenly trying to build herself a little more firmly into my next book.

"A long wait indeed", I rejoined, "but one that I was fairly relaxed about, because, in Gatwick there is a very fine Champagne and Seafood Bar into which I was comfortably ensconced before the clock struck ten"

"Basil, is this relevant?" she interrupted.

"I will let you be the judge of that" I said, and continued. I had just a half bottle of champagne, to start, scrambled eggs and smoked salmon, whilst reflecting on the life of a celebrity" I smiled. She frowned. Before the clock had struck the half hour, I had both drunken and eaten. There was still over four hours to kill, so I had a little wander. I resisted the urge to pay £70 for a ticket to win a Bentley. I narrowly avoided a credit card that would enable me to have naught per-cent interest on all Balance Transfers for one year, and then I………."

"Basil" the ice was forming again.

"Sorry" I murmured, but I wasn't really. "Anyway, 2.30 arrived, by which time I had probably quaffed another half a glass of bubbly, and so I set off for Gate 39". She breathed a sigh of relief that I had a least got down off the bar stool. "I have had, for many years," I continued, reacting to her evident relief, a little fold-up trolley on wheels onto which I can put a small bag. So, I put my small bag on the little fold-up trolley on wheels, and set off for Gate 39. To reach the gate I had to descend a very long escalator, and I athletically hopped on to the top step whilst dexterously swinging my little fold-up trolley on wheels to land beside me. Sadly, my little fold-up trolley on wheels, had lost the plot. It folded up *prematurely*, leaving my little non-folding bag unrestrained thus enabling it, quite unexpectedly to catapult itself between my ankles, causing me, in geometrical terms, to describe a perfect arc, before, I am told, landing head first on the third step down and then continuing base over apex to the bottom" I avoided the anatomically equivalent description, and paused for a moment to let her take in this intriguing scene. She took in the intriguing scene.

"You tripped over your bag" she said in a voice that took all of the adventure out, and made it sound like a clumsy accident. I ignored her and continued

"I awoke some minutes later in the Ladies Loo with a face, neck and shirt covered in blood, two delightful hostesses sponging me off, and a paramedic, trying to persuade me to let him stitch up my ear." I waited for a comment, but beyond a resigned sigh, Nita was po-faced. "Anyway, to cut a long story short"

"Harrumph" came from the chair the other side of the desk, but I continued.

"To cut a long story short, the hostesses explained that I appeared to have knocked myself out when I landed on my head, and had spent the rest of the journey from the top to the bottom of the escalator oblivious of the passengers I had probably bowled over, if not bowled out". A wry smile played around Nita's lips. "Champagne, of course, had no part in this absurd attention grab" she mumbled. I ignored her, but not her comment.

"They did, of course, satisfy themselves that I was neither tired, nor emotional, and that my longish stay at the champagne and seafood bar had more to do with the quality of the Whitstable oysters, than the quantity of the house champagne. The paramedic put away his needle and thread, and the two hostesses escorted me to the aircraft, jumping the queue, and *mentally* upgrading me to *notional* business class, (a seat in row one which usually requires an '*extra legroom*' premium) and attended to my every need for the next four hours. Once more I reflected on the life of a celebrity". I leaned back in the chair expecting her to applaud the agility that had succeeded in getting me a *notional* upgrade. There was a flicker of amusement, and I guessed the warm glow was back.

"I expect you want to know where the clot came in." I asked, warming to my story.

"I know exactly where he came in" she said"; he came in through the door in the corner of my room". She pointed, and to show how much I valued her tit for tat repartee, I said,

"Nita, you are a star".

"And you, Basil" she said, "are a danger to the public who should not be let out without a minder"

"Will you be my minder?" I replied quickly, knowing that I had made her an offer she could not refuse. She refused with the rather unnecessary retort.

"I would rather poke myself in the eye with a sharp stick" but now her eyes were twinkling and I knew that our old rapport had been regained. She continued, semi-serious now. "Basil, you *are* an enigma, I love listening to you, but, it is late, I have a husband, I have two children, I want to see them, and they want to see me, so, please, tell me what you want".

"Well Nita, putting aside my little finger, my thumb, my badly sunburned lip and my suspected hernia..........I think my cancer might be returning for the third time, and, despite the fact that I always appear to take life lightly, I do, as you know, have my Tigers, (*see AND THE TIGERS*

COME AT NIGHT) and they have been giving me a hard time lately.

"Tell me about the blood clot?" she said

"clots" I replied, "there were two of them. The Gatwick escalator may be involved"

"How?".

"Well", after I got to Tenerife my left hand was giving me quite a lot of pain and I could not move my little finger"

"Was it broken?"

"Well, that is what I thought, and on the Friday Polly told me that I had finally decided to go to the Hospital A&E to get an X-Ray".

"And?"

"And I ended up as their guest for five days, during which time they decided that the tendon to my little finger had snapped and could now be anywhere between the palm of the hand and the Ascension Islands" I looked at her

"So you did what?" she asked.

"So, I stayed in the hospital until they gave me their prognosis and explained the *'hunt the tendon'* procedure, and then discharged myself deciding I would rather have a stiff little finger than scars and stitches all over my hand, and half way up my arm."

"I follow all this Basil, BUT" she drummed her fingers on the table "what about the blood clots?"

"I'm just coming to that" I said

"And I'm just waiting for you to come to that" she retorted.

"OK. Well you see, my hand was still very painful, and now my right thumb was also, not only giving a lot of pain, but periodically kept locking. On the advice of a friend I went to a para-farmacist and got a bottle of 60 tablets called *Vitameal-Artrin* at a cost of 28 euros, for one month's supply, so they had to be good. Anyway, everybody promised that they would take the pain away, and I would suffer no side effects."

"OK, then what?"

"On the first day I took two with breakfast, from then on, all through the day I kept feeling that I wanted to wee, except I couldn't manage it. By the evening, I had so much pain in my groin area that I ended up kneeling on the settee in the lounge to try and relieve it. Then I went to the loo again and forced and forced and got a tiny dribble that was clearly coloured by blood. And then a small clot appeared, very small, almost minute. The pain persisted. I went to a restaurant with the family that evening, and could hardly sit still, I paid two or three visits down a long flight of stairs to the gents, and then, on the third, a much larger blood clot appeared and I was able to wee freely. No blood in the flow. That was five or six weeks ago, and since then I have had the occasional return of the pain, and several more small blood clots". I looked at her with my serious face "That's why I'm here Nita"

"You shouldn't have left it so long Basil"

"I know, but if I spent five days in the Green Hospital for a stiff little finger, I thought they might give me life if I went back with a blood clot".

"Basil, what can I do for you?"

"Well, I suppose I want a bit of comfort, I suppose I want you to say...'*Don't worry about that blood clot Basil, it's probably just something you've eaten*'. I suppose I want you to say, *"No Basil, it's quite OK, the cancer hasn't come back'* I suppose....."

"Basil" quietly now, concerned, the Nita I really know "Lets get some blood now, I'll get it off to the lab, and we can see what's happening to the PSA, we can also make a few other tests, Don't let's pre-judge anything, there are numerous reasons that can account for what has happened."

She smiled, and so did I, I felt better already. "I'll just phone home" she said, and tell them I will be a little while, and whilst we are sorting things out you can bring me up to date with everything that has happened since the cancer returned last time".

Nita went out to make her call, and I began to get my thoughts in order for when she came back.

It was just 33 months since Nita first spotted my cancer, and 29 months since Mr. Breading had taken his knife to my prostate.

CHAPTER 1

IMPLANTS RE-VISTED

If there is anybody out there who read the first of my reflections on '*My Tigers*', they may recall that *Book 1* ended, some months after the operation to remove my prostate, with the vision of a highly re-trained athlete coming to grips (if you will forgive the expression) with the wonderful world of vacuum pumps, Viagra, Levitra, Ciallis, and Muse. Though stopping just short of direct injections, implants and even transplants.

In the months that followed, I threw myself into a radical re-training of all I had ever been taught about bedroom athletics. No test was to stiff *(it was generally **only** the tests that were)* and I practiced whenever I had a spare moment, *(and of course a willing partner)*. I gave new meaning to the word improvisation, and for much of the time I was rewarded by a *very* smiley face *(usually mine)*. I would, no longer be considered a player of county standard *(if indeed I ever had been)*, but, at club level I would have been rated as a good trier with an innovative, if somewhat unusual style. But, whilst I have never quite mastered the art of breathing through my ears, I felt that perhaps I was earning a C+ in the satisfaction department, even though I definitely did not need a stone in my shoe to make me limp. I often remembered Mr. Breading's pre-op pep talk.

"If **we** are lucky I will manage to remove the prostate **without** damaging the nerves that enable you to stand up for yourself"

Well, **he** may have been lucky and is probably still a regular *'stand-up'* guy, but to quote a good old *school-boy* joke, *(yes, I was a school boy once) 'I may still have twelve inches, but I don't use it as a rule'.*

From this point on, the chapter is not for the faint-hearted so please feel free to skip forward to where I begin to rip apart Einstien's theories on both quantum physics and relativity.

I recalled an earlier visit to Mr. Breading when he had posed the question. "Basil, and tell me about your love life",

I had, in the rush to make my point, told him about how helpful the internet had been on the subject of penile implants. At that time he had mumbled *(that's why it's in smaller print)* something about

"Far too early, looking over the brink, give it another few months, don't do them myself. Have a colleague in Leicester who does," and finally "So tell me Basil, what you think of this new lad Freddie Flintoff". I had gathered from that that the subject was closed, if not totally taboo. In any event, I had given it another few months, but I felt, the time was now right to try to make the acquaintance of this *'colleague in Leicester'* As I prepared therefore to give him a call to arrange a special introductory consultation, I boned up on my subject.

"I will go" I said to Polly, one Gin and Tonic drinking

evening at the Lime Tree Restaurant, *(I had never felt the same about Kir Royale since Alison (Book 1) had told me about the table wine code for hospital weeing)* "to the public library and read up all I can about Penile Implants"

"That's a good idea" said Polly, "but why don't you just look on the internet first?"

"What a good idea" I responded, recognizing, as always, a good idea whenever Polly told me she had just had one.

"And where" I started smugly "do you suggest I can look?" I gave her a superior, not to say imperious gaze down my nose, knowing that she knew very little about computers.

"Why don't you Google it?" said Polly.

Now then, knowing as I have said, that Polly's knowledge of the internet is akin with my knowledge of housework, I could only assume that, in one of her magazines there had been a *'letter to Mary'* along the lines of.

Dear Mary,
We have been married 7 years
And my husband Bert doesn't
seem interested any more….
What can I do?
Frustrated of Scunthorpe

Dear Frustrated of Scunthorpe.
Why don't you tell him to Google it?

"Well," I said, "I've tried everything else so I'll give it a go" I looked at her with my head on one side "two questions….*first* what do I have to do?, *second,* does it hurt? and *third*, who the hell has been teaching you such bizarre sexual practices as Googling?"

"You said two questions" said Polly ever calm "but to answer all three, *first*, you have to enter the key word into

3

the little box at the top of your computer screen….the one marked 'Google' *second*, for what you were just thinking I jolly well hope it does hurt, and *third* Mr. Partington at number 38." Suddenly I knew she was joking……………... Mr. Partington lives at No. 34.

I Googled it.

IMPLANTS It said

Do you mean….DENTAL/BREAST/HAIR

I then tried. **PENILE IMPLANTS.** It said

Sorry, no matches for …IMPLpENILE IMPLANTS ….try again

I tried again, taking a little more care with my spelling. Now, from this point on, Gentlemen get your pencils sharpened, and Ladies, put your glasses on. But for the squeamishly repressed, please skip a couple of pages. The search came back….and I quote.

<u>Make your Penis Bigger.</u>

<u>Viagra users beware</u>

<u>Improve Penile function</u>

<u>Penile Implants for Erection Problems</u>

And finally, the one I wanted.

<u>Penile Implants, What to Expect and How to prepare</u>

I clicked the link and read eagerly. Let me share what I found, because Gentlemen, the need for excitement may have become a thing of the past, and Ladies, you could have just found the PERFECT Christmas present for the *'man who has **almost** everything'*.

Penile Implants, What to Expect and How to prepare

Penile implants can reduce erectile dysfunction. EXPLORE your choices and find out what to expect from this special procedure.

Penile implants are artificial devices implanted inside the penis that allow men with erectile dysfunction (ED) to achieve an erection instantly. There are TWO basic designs.

INFLATABLE. *Also called hydraulic. Inflatable implants can be pumped up to create an erection and then deflated*

SEMI-RIGID. *These implants are permanently,* **somewhat,** *firm.*

The web site ran to seven pages, all of which I printed off to read, and re-read at my leisure. It included, diagrams and pictures, and an eventual itinerary for approximately £7,000 well spent.

Travel to the Czech Republic *(in the UK it is much more expensive)* Accommodation for eight to nine days, food, if you felt like it, and pre and post consultations included.

Polly thought I was mad….but I quite liked the prospect of 'instant control' Two squeezes for **Yes Please,** One squeeze, for **'I've got one of your old headaches'** After several millennium, man could get his own back and say **'I don't want'** without nature giving him away.

'Sorry dear, I'd love to, but my squeegee appears to be stuck'

One element worried me. And I discussed it over a number of emails exchanged with the clinic in Prague. However, I was almost ready to go, when the events later described in this book put all such thoughts on hold as bigger priorities took over. So what was that worrying element? Let me quote from one of the emails received in the middle of the summer 2006, and at the point where I was about to send the Czech a Cheque.

The operation, although both complex and permanent, has become relatively common since being first introduced in the

1970's. New materials, designs, and surgical procedures have greatly improved outcomes for penile implants. Most men who have the procedure AND their partners say they are more than satisfied with the results.

No worries there then…but here it comes.

After your stay in our clinic, you will receive the very best of post operative care. We will then make an appointment for you to return approximately 5 weeks after surgery for an examination…….

Wait for it, because I kid you not.

*After the operation the device will be left **INFLATED** and must remain so until your final examination in 5 weeks. Please ensure that you have with you LOOSE UNDERWEAR, (Boxer shorts preferred) because, effectively, you will have a permanent erection until your return. It is advised that you partake in no sexual activity until after this time.*

Now, the way I see it you would be partaking in sexual activity every time you bent down to tie your shoe lace, but what do I know? Enough to say that I was *not* deterred because the pluses seemed to outweigh the minuses. Czech Republic here I come….except that I didn't, at least, not then.

Before I could make an appointment to go to Prague, I received a phone call from Georgina, Mr. B's secretary. "Mr. Jay" she said, "Mr. Breading wonders if you could pop in and see him?" I was slightly taken aback.

"Well, yes", I said slowly,

"Do you know why?"

"I'm afraid not" she said sweetly, "but he did ask me to

ask you if you could make it as soon as possible?" she paused, and before I could answer, said "Perhaps Friday morning at 11.30".

"Thank you Georgina" I said, "please tell Mr. B. I will be there"

The next day or two passed very slowly and I quietly put my Penile Implant information into my sock drawer.

CHAPTER 2

EARWIG OH AGAIN

"Sit there Basil" I sat there. The nurse had pointed at a very small, overstuffed easy chair against the wall, an overstuffed chair that an overstuffed backside would render overcrowded. I rendered it overcrowded. "Mr. Breading will be back in a Jiffy" For a fleetingly flippant moment I was tempted to ask whether he would be wearing it or driving it, but for once, although the nurse was possessed of a face that could, as Homer would have said, '*have launched a thousand quips*', I, the redoubtable Basil Jay, was in a particularly un-quipable mood.

"Thank you" I said instead. She left. I stayed. I looked around the small but comfortable consulting room, and then out of the small window upon the wind-blown December car park. It wanted just 3 days to Christmas Day 2006, and I was feeling decidedly un-Christmassy.

"Basil" boomed a voice from the doorway behind me, I recognized the timbre in the voice of the only man to have ever held my unprotected prostate in his gloved hand, "so tell me, how are you?" Before I could turn around to face him he had circled the room, rounded his desk, angled his square, well built frame on to his chair, and steepled his fingers. He looked at me, and I realized it was going to be a very geometric sort of a day. I prised my over-stuffed backside out of the over-stuffed easy chair and sat in the uncomfortable looking wheel-back in front of his desk. I looked for his Jiffy; he was neither wearing it nor driving it. He must have left it in the corridor.

"I feel fine" I said "in myself".

How stupid is that response that we often give when we are not 100%, what an earth does it mean. I feel fine...*in myself,* does that mean that you feel pretty groggy...*outside of yourself,* and decidedly unwell in *anybody else.* However, I did not share these thoughts with the Great Man, but merely continued with. "Of course, I am a bit apprehensive, that you have had your secretary call me to ask if I could just 'Pop In'". I looked into his eyes as I said "It sounds a little bit ominous."

"Ahhh" he said

"Ummmm" I replied

"I was a bit concerned" he said, "about your recent blood test. I have a copy of it here" he waved a piece of paper in the air in case I didn't believe him.

"Ahhh" I said

"Ummmm" he replied

"Your PSA is 0.2"

"Ahhh" I said, and before he could even think about his Ummmm, continued "that's OK isn't it?"

"Ummmm" he said, obviously determined not to be out-Ahhhhhed. "When you have a prostrate it is fine, but without a prostrate................Ummmm" He let the sentence tail into nothingness, waiting for my response.

"Ahhh" I said, predictably

"Ummm" he replied. "You see, it has gone from 0.1 to 0.2 since your last test, that is less than one month", *(he didn't enquire why I had arranged two blood tests so close together, and I didn't enlighten him that the second had supposed to be for cholesterol but I had taken the wrong form)* and that indicates that it is just possible," he paused before repeating "***just*** possible, that we may have left a bit of cell tissue behind" Hey, wait a minute, my mind cried out, what's all this ***we*** business, I just lay on table there dreaming of my favourite car park attendant *(See AND THE TIGERS COME AT NIGHT)* . You were the one wielding the knife. However, I said nothing, so he carried on, briskly "BUT, no reason for us to get despondent, it may just be a rogue reading. When are you going back to Tenerife?" I thought he was changing the subject.

"Well", I said, I am taking the whole family, ten of us, ski-ing the week after Christmas. We get back from France on the 14th of January, and plan to go back to the sun a few days after that"

"Ahhhh" he said

"Ummmmm" I replied

"Rightho" he looked me in the eye, "please do me a favour first". "I'll try" I said

"Pop in here as soon as you get back" he opened his diary "say on the 15th, and have them do a blood test, and then come and see me the following day, on the 16th."

"Alright" I said, I wanted to ask him if I had a real problem, but couldn't quite find the words. "See my secretary, Georgina, on the way out and she will make the appointments. Tell her to make sure she squeezes you in even if I have a full appointments book." I had started to rise from the chair when, as if reading my unspoken words, he said, "I don't want you to worry about this Basil"

"I'll try not to" I said as I reached the door.

"Good" he said "good, good , good, good"

I closed the door, but the *'goods'* followed me into the

corridor, I was careful not to trip over his Jiffy, but it was nowhere to be seen. I made my arrangements with Georgina and left. As I walked to the car I spoke silently to my Tigers. "Well chaps" I said, "Earwig oh again"

Chapter 3

DIVER TICKLE ME WHAT?
(JANUARY 2007)

You may remember my Tigers, my nocturnal friends, my pre-dawn patrol. There were four of them.

__FEAR__....who always burst into my mind unbidden with unsheathed claws, bared teeth and a roar like the Victoria Falls. He was always so negative, so pessimistic, two traits that scared the life out of me, but, at the same time made me angry. That anger had got me through many a nasty night when the curtain had first risen on __Basil's Prostate Path ....Act One.__ And then there was

__HOPE...__a pussy cat, who nuzzled into the mind and calmed the anger, and said everything would be alright. Hope, who made the dawn seem closer and the day that followed brighter.

__Fear__ and __Hope__ were my main companions, busier when the day's news had been bad, quietly patrolling the peripheries of my mind when a day passed without news good or bad. I had two more Tigers, infrequent visitors, who came only when the advice of Fear or Hope had failed to sustain me. I called *them **Regret** and **Resignation.** But they were just bit players who contributed nothing of a positive nature in a drama that had to be played out by just the three of us. **Basil,** his **Fear** and his **Hope.***

I returned from my rare *solo* visit to Mr. Breading and Polly brought me a small Gin and Tonic in a bucket and said "What was it all about?" I told her "Oh" she said, ever pragmatic

"Oh indeed" I replied, ever perceptive.

"You're spilling your drink" she answered, ever practical. "You did make the appointments didn't you?" she got out her diary. I got out the little appointment card that Georgina had given me. – at least, I would have done if I could have found it.

"I must have left in the garage when I paid for the petrol" I said, "because I had it in my wallet, and I couldn't find my credit card and so I had to take a few things out of my wallet whilst I was looking for it and I must hav……"

"I'll phone and check" she said breaking into my ramblings.

"There's no need" I replied, "I *know* it was 9.30 am on the 15th January for the blood test, and 12.30 on the 16th January for the audience with the Great Man" she phoned anyway.

"Your blood test is 12.30 on the 15th " she told me ten minutes later, "and your appointment with Mr. B is at 9.30 on the 16th"

"Ouch" I said

"Take your feet off the sofa" she replied

"OK" said Polly "it's in my diary, so now just forget about it and let's plan Christmas for the three of us". The

matter was closed, and self pity was simply not allowed....
quite right too,

"Right ho" I said, but I knew that would be having a
little chat with my Tiger friends when the rest of the world
was asleep.

Count down, two days to Christmas. I had had an
easy night, my Tigers had visited, but ***Hope*** had been the
dominant one *"Basil," he had said "Mr. B got it right, it is
obviously just a rogue reading...anyway, he told you not to
worry, and you promised him you wouldn't.....done deal, go
to sleep and plan Christmas and the ski-ing."*

Fear *tried to get a look in...."Ahhhh" he said, Mr. B may
be wrong, and waiting almost a month seems a bit foolhardy
to me, if the cancer is back and it is growing, a lot can happen
in a month" But his usual roar, was nothing more than an
irritating growl.*

"Sod off" I said, and off he sodded.

Polly and I sat down to a boiled egg and a pot of tea
and coffee and planned our very quiet Christmas. "Did you
sleep well?" Polly asked

"Like a top" I answered, wondering at the same time
what an earth a 'top' sleeps like, and anyway, what the
hell is a 'top'. A bit of philosophy for another day. We were
going to be three for Christmas because we have had this
arrangement with our children ever since they got themselves
'significant others',

'significant others', who, I must now say, have become
two wives and a husband. The arrangement is, that they all
spend Christmas with their spouses families one Christmas,
and they, all six of them (now seven with additions) spend
the alternate Christmas with us. So this year was the In-Law
Christmas, and so we were three for Christmas lunch, just
Polly, myself and my mother *(the Tigers were not invited).*

"Why don't we" said Polly, "go to the Lime Tree on Christmas Eve?" Polly is unfortunate to have a birthday on Christmas Eve which means she has always been a little short-changed on celebrations, "and then have a quiet Christmas Dinner at home"

"That sounds fine to me" I said, and the phone rang. Polly picked it up. I can always tell which of our three children are on the phone by the way Polly answers it "Hi Tim" half an Octave above the norm and rising, unsurprisingly means it's Tim on the phone "Hello Lou Lou" with Lou Lou pitched a tone below Hello means it's my daughter Tania, and "It's me" almost in a whisper means it's our youngest, Jeremy, who always says into the phone as soon as it is picked up "It's Me" to which Polly simply replies "It's me"

Polly picked up the phone, a heartbeat passed, and then "it's me", followed by, "Oh that's a nice surprise, followed by "looooverly" followed by "see you tomorrow then" She put down the phone and smiled, "Guess what?" she said.

"Jem and Steph are joining us for Christmas Eve" I said

"Yessss" she said,

"I better make it FIVE at the Lime Tree." The phone rang. Polly picked it up.

"Hello Lou Lou – how are you? are you? When? Where? all of you? Tomorrow? with James and Margot? oh that will be loooooverly, how's Jack? how's Nigel? what time? The ferry or the train? yes that's better, what time? for lunch? See you tomorrow then, byeeee" Polly looked across at me. "Guess what?" I was getting good at this and said.

"Tania, Nigel, and Jack are coming tomorrow by ferry or train, probably ferry because they will be in the car, because they are going to spend Christmas day at Surbiton with James and family, mum and dad are traveling up from

15

York, and so they want to spend Christmas Eve with us to celebrate your birthday".

"More or less" said Polly

"Well, I said, we better do a birthday lunch, because they won't want to be too late away if they are going to Surbiton, and anyway, lunch is much better for Jack" I would have carried on, but the phone rang. Polly picked it up

"Hi Tim, you're back, did you have a good time? not there for Christmas, poor girl, lates, that's unlucky, no we'd love to see you, tomorrow, about twelve…that's loooooverly, I will have you all here for my birthday. Yes, Jem and Steph are coming, and Nigel Tania and Jack on their way from Paris to Surbiton, yes, with James and Margot, I understand that they are coming up form York; yes there will be a house full. OK, see you tomorrow morning. Yes Granny will be here, she's getting a an early train to Ashford and Dad is picking her up at about 10.30, look forward to it. Byeee"

She didn't say, guess what, but this time I had a question.

"Tim and Vee are supposed to be in Helsinki, what's happened?" My daughter in-law is Finnish and their plan had been Christmas in Finland with her family.

"Well, apparently she has to work on Boxing Day (Vee is a forensic scientist with the Metropolitan Police) and her work rota has been changed. They didn't tell us in advance in case things changed, but they got back from Helsinki last night and would like to spend Christmas with us. My boiled Egg was cold

I booked the Harrow for ten people and we had a splendid Christmas Eve, birthday lunch full of chatter and crackers and funny hats. The boys stayed for Christmas Day, and surprise surprise, Tania Nigel and Jack were able to call in for another couple of days on their way back to Paris. Christmas drew to a close, and we were just a few days from meeting up again in Chamonix for a week's ski-ing......or so we thought.

The air tickets were booked and paid for, the chalet was booked and paid for, it was the 4th of January and in just 3 days time we would be on the piste.....or so we thought. But there was one of life's little surprises awaiting us. On the night of the 4th, Polly felt a little unwell, as it was stomach cramps she assumed it was over indulgence at Christmas. She woke up in the morning pale and wan *(I've always wanted to say that)* she got no better as the day progressed and so we made an appointment for her to go see the doctor. He was unable to help very much but, as it was approaching the week-end, suggested that if she was no better she should go the A&E at Maidstone Hospital. She wasn't. So we did. After an interminably long wait and a thorough examination I was sent home to get her a little goody bag because they had decided to admit her for tests. I didn't argue, but went home and collect for her a dressing gown, half a pair of slippers *(I don't know what happened to the other half)* a tube of toothpaste a toothbrush, and I couldn't think of anything else. When I got back she had been admitted to a ward, and I went down to the hospital shop to buy a comb. I explained that I couldn't see any of the dozen or so she said we had at home. On the way down I had the chance to ask the doctor what was wrong.

"*Diver tickle me ivories*" he said, obviously mistaking me for some under-water piano player, hired to provide the Hospital's Christmas Panto.

"I'm sorry" I said

"I think she has what we call *diver tickle me ivories*" he said, but we do want to run some test to be sure what we are dealing with" It was Friday night.

"We are supposed to be flying to Geneva on Tuesday" I

said, "for the start of a family ski-ing holiday. Had I better cancel the flight?"

"Let's wait and see what Monday brings" he said, and it was clear that the interview was over. I went and sat by Polly's bedside.

"I've just spoken to the doctor" I said, "he seems to think it's not serious, just something called '*diver tickle me ivories*'"

"called what?" said Polly.

"*Diver tickle me ivories* – yes stupid name isn't it, probably called after some African Witch Doctor"

"*Diverticulitis*" said a voice behind me

"Sorry" I turned around and there was a pretty black nurse smiling broadly

"It is called *Diverticulitis*" she repeated with a smile, "and as far as I know it was NOT discovered by an African Witch Doctor." She could hardly suppress her mirth. "But once I tell them in the common room about *Diver tickle me ivories,* I think it might just catch on." Whether it did or not I will never know, what I do know is that that little nurse was a treasure; she tried her best to get Polly out of hospital in time for the Tuesday flight, but to no avail. It did turn out to be Diverticulitis and no treatment was necessary. But by the time the doctors had made that decision Tuesday had been and gone and went, so we had to re-book our flights for the Thursday, thus losing two days of our seven, *(to say nothing of the cost of the Tuesday flight)* but at least when we arrived at our quite splendid chalet, the garden of which opened directly on to the piste, the children had got everything organized. The fridge was stocked, the wine racks were full, and skis and boots were ready in the hall.

As this is not a book about ski-ing but the inner workings of the body and that grand institution called hospital, I will not spend any time on the ski-ing other to say, it was a wonderful week, we arrived back without any broken bones. And we had watched our grandson Jack, just short of his third birthday; take to the slopes on skis as only the very young can.

CHAPTER 4

CURTAIN UP.....ACT TWO
(JANUARY 2007)

The Winterlands car park is becoming as familiar to me as my own driveway. And it was with a feeling of De Ja Vue that I parked outside the front entrance at 9.30 on the 16th January and prepared to throw my car keys to a waiting porter. Sadly there was not one in attendance. As in fact there had not been the previous day when I had arrived for my blood test.

I sauntered in as if I did not have a care in the world and threw a careless "Hello Georgie" to Mr. Breading's secretary, she caught it and replied with a stern face,

"Hello Mr. Jay", nice to see you again..........and it's Georgina – by the way"

"Sorry" I said, even though I wasn't, "it's nice to see you again, although it's not nice to be back" I paused, to let my grin slide across my face and then said "and it's Basil – by the way" She laughed, the stern fell off her face, and we were friends again.

"Mr. Breading is in conference with one of his colleagues,

but he won't be long. If you sit outside his room you will see him walk down the corridor." Ah, *walk*, I reflected, he must have sold his Jiffy.

Sure enough, I had no sooner opened the July 1993 edition of House and Garden *(this time Polly was with me)* and she had managed to grab the more up to date 1997 version, when he came striding along.

"Basil" he boomed, "and Mrs. Jay, follow me" We followed him:

"do come in" he held the door open for us and, ignoring the chair that I had over-crowded on my own, on the last visit, Polly and I made straight for the rickety wheel backs in front of his desk. "How was the ski-ing?" he asked as soon as he had sat down. Why oh why do they do that? The dentist always wants to know where you are going for your holidays just seconds after he has thrust his fingers down your throat. The hairdresser wants to know if you saw last nights Panorama seconds after she has plunged your head into six inches of luke warm water, and the consultant wants to know how you enjoyed the ski-ing when all you want to know is whether you'll be alive next Tuesday.

"Most enjoyable" I said, playing the game according to the script, and going on to tell him all about Polly's diverticulitis and Jack's ski-ing prowess at just 3 years old, all the time wondering what my PSA now was. Eventually, he looked serious.

"It's now up to 0.4 he said without further pre-amble, and so I have taken the liberty of discussing your case with Mr. Draper. Harry Draper is the consultant radiologist. He would like to see you before you go back to Tenerife. Is that possible?"

"Of course" I said, "we have no commitments that we can't change. When does he want to see me?"

"Now," he said, he has a clinic today, he is just down the

corridor, and he told me to wheel you along as soon as I had finished with you" Wheel me along, I thought, perhaps he hasn't sold his Jiffy after all.

"That's fine", I said, "Can you tell me just what this increase to 0.4 means?"

"I could" he said, "but as I am handing you over to Mr. Draper, it might be better if he explains".

"OK" I said, somewhat weakly, reflecting that Mr. B had just earned a pretty easy £90, and whether I had learned enough yet to become a geriatric prostate consultant.

Mr. Breading almost frog-marched us along the corridor, and without a knock ushered us into the presence of Mr. Harry Draper who was as different to Mr. B as two men could be. He was probably late thirties, tall and slim with a very intellectual look. He was wearing a very smart chalk striped suit and a silk tie. Whereas Mr. B conjured up a picture of muddy rugger pitches, grubby knees, and un-protected prostates, Dr. D projected a mental image of careful thought. You could almost see his long fingers stroking his Bishop, or coaxing his Jack out of the pack as he faced a protagonist across the chess board or the Bridge table.

"Harry, this is Basil and his wife Anne" boomed Mr. B, I've briefed them about our chat, so over to you" and he was gone – or almost, at the door, as if a thought had struck him, he paused, looked over his shoulder, and said "You know where I am if you want me Basil, but for now you are in good hands" and then he was gone….completely.

Dr. Draper stood up and leaned over his desk with his hand outstretched, he smiled, and raised an eyebrow as if to say 'with Mr. B your feet don't touch the ground' he didn't, but he did say, "Hello Mr. Jay, Mrs. Jay, it's nice to meet you both and Mr. Breading has told me all about your case." I was immediately put at ease, and felt that I could be pretty direct with this man.

"It's nice to meet you Dr. Draper" he smiled, "I have to say that Mr. Breading has told me very little about the happenings of the last couple of months…I hope you can explain a few things to me"

"Of course I can, and I will" he said "but perhaps I should first of all explain the difference between myself and Mr. Breading, and why he has reluctantly given up your company" I was warming to this man.

"I am, of course a doctor, but my specialisation is Radiology and associated cancer treatments. To put it bluntly, Mr. B wields the knife, but I prefer to fight cancers without surgery, where that is an option", I sort of nodded wondering why I hadn't gone to him in the first place, then I remembered how Mr. B had spelled out all the options for me very clearly and carefully, and how, although he recommended surgery, it had been my ultimate decision.

Dr. D was continuing. "Surgery is no longer necessary for you, nor in fact is it an option, because, although you don't need reminding, your prostate has already been removed." He paused to let me catch up. I caught up. "Now I know that Mr. Breading would have explained that, even after a radical prostatectomy, there are sometimes small pieces of cancerous tissue left behind. Sometimes in-fact the cancer has already spread to the lymph nodes. We measure the chances of this happening by monitoring your PSA levels. Your reading should remain at a constant level below 0.1… and so it did for a full year. However, in November it had crept up to 0.2 and that was why Mr. Breading asked to see you and had you take another blood test. I have that result now, I am afraid it has risen again to 0.4." He paused yet again so that I could take it all in. I took it all in. "However, it is not time to panic, but it is time to investigate. What I would like to do therefore is to arrange for you to have a full body bone scan and an MRI so that we can see exactly what is happening. I then want to give it 3 or 4 more weeks and take another PSA reading. Depending on the results of those three tests we can decide what treatment is appropriate"

"What do you think it is likely to be?" I asked him, a little nervously.

"I am not going to pre-judge" he smiled, "but I will tell you this, a PSA of 0.4 is still low, what is more worrying is the rate of increase. This would suggest that there is a little cancerous tissue left there and it is growing fairly quickly. We must be sure of where it is before I can decide on the treatment"

"What are the choices?" I asked.

"Well, there are several, in view of what you have already been through, I would imagine that we will probably be looking at Hormone Therapy, Chemo Therapy and Radio Therapy ...all, or just some of them" he smiled again "but let's do no guessing, let's just get the tests organized." What more was there for me to say?

"We are due to go back to Tenerife in a day or so" I did say, "if you don't want to see me until then can we go ahead with that, I will of course fly back whenever I have to".

"Yes, that's fine" he said, "but I would like to set up all the appointments now, and you can then treat your return to Tenerife as a short holiday rather than a return to your winter home" He leaned forward and put his elbows on the desk. "Basil, what is happening to you is worrying, but a long long way from serious. It is now the 16th January. You go off to Tenerife now and my secretary Jo will make all the arrangements and email you" he stopped as if a sudden idea had struck him "you do have email in Tenerife I suppose?"

"Oh absolutely" I said, "and running water, and electricity, and even an inside toilet." He laughed, and

I laughed...the first from each of us during the whole consultation.

"We will give you a bit of notice, but I would think we would be looking at the middle of February – how is that for you?"

"That's just fine" I said "Can you tell me, will I be seeing other doctors now or just you?"

"Well, of course, that is up to you, but I have all of your case notes and I would be very happy to take things from here, if you are happy with that"

"Dr. Draper" I said, "I feel very comfortable with that and I will certainly not be consulting anybody else."

We all stood up and shook hands. I will see you in three or four weeks"

As we walked through the now deserted corridor, I remembered my promise not to consult anybody else. I knew that that was not strictly true, because from today on I knew I would be having nightly consultations with my Tigers.

Chapter 5

AKA DOLLY PARTON
(FEBRUARY 2007)

Just like the first time around, I was able to have a serious talk with my Tigers and tell them to leave me alone until they really had something to worry me about…..and they did. We found that we could not quite get back into our usual winter round of golfing delights. Which will be fully explained to my golfing friends if I simply refer to No Swallow's, No Taboo's and definitely No Scramble's. At least we played in them, but in the knowledge that we were possibly going to be there for only a week or two for the rest of the winter, our hearts were not in the competitions. True to his word, I received an email from Dr. D's secretary Jo, informing me that she had made appointments for an MRI scan (3rd Sunday in February) a full body bone scan, (the following Tuesday), a blood test (the same day) and an appointment with Dr. D for the Friday following, The die, was cast. We flew home on the Friday before the MRI scan and I went through the same procedure that I described in Tigers 1. But not quite. Though the procedure was the same the venue was different. The first time I had had my MRI in the comfort of the state of the art new oncology wing of Maidstone Hospital. This time I had it in the car park at Winterlands. Last time it was a beautiful late summer day in early September. This time it was brass monkey with knobs on, or nearly not, depending which way you look at it. Last time I had worn a blue gown and pretty blue over slippers as I walked through the centrally heated corridors of the architects dream. This time I still wore the blue gown, but this time I had on my street shoes and no socks as I walked across the gravel car park to the mobile unit. BUT, once in the warmth of said caravan, the girls were lovely, the treatment was thorough *(I lay under the scanner for more than three quarters of an hour),* and was let back out into the February car park with the reassuring words

"We will make sure that Dr. Draper has got these in good time for your consultation," a pause whilst she looked at her notes, "next Friday". I gave them a cherry wave, fell down the steps of the caravan, and described my length *(as we pretentious novelists say)* upon the ground of the car park, so crisp and steep and uneven, that it could still have been Christmas. Before they could rush to my assistance, I sprung to my feet, and with a grimaced "Whoops" went back to the warmth of the hospital and my clothes.

Two days later I was in the hospital for the body scan, and this really did follow the same procedure, in the same place, by the same operator *(who, as a matter of interest, did NOT recognize me from my previous visit).* I reminded her of our late night assignation almost 18 month earlier. The empty hospital, her words of comfort, and her heartfelt good wishes. She immediately said, "Ah, of course I remember you **Bryan**". I didn't pursue it, because at least she had said it the posh way.....with a y.

There was an interesting footnote to this particular test. I telephoned Jo *(Dr. D's secretary you will remember)* on the morning of my consultation, just to make sure that he had the scans.

"We do have a slight problem Mr. Jay" she said, "the scans are ready, but are still at Maidstone General. Is there any chance that you could pick them up and bring them with you when you come, and give them to reception so Dr. Draper has time to study them before he sees you?"

"That's fine" I said, "will they give them to me?"

"I'll phone them and tell them to expect you" she said. And so, with Polly driving I called in at Oncology, was directed to the Nuclear Science Dept, told them the reason for my visit, and was told to sit quietly and the prints would be read in a tick. I waited for more ticks than you need to get an O level in an 'ology, and then poked my head around the door of the little room where about 500 doctors, nurses and porters seemed to be congregated.

"Harumph" I cleared my throat, "I was wondering whether the results of my body scan are ready yet, as I have an appointment over at Winterlands with Dr. D. shortly and he wants me to take them with me."

"Name" said a gruff speaking older man.

"Basil Jay" I said

"Jay" he said, "Jay, Jay, Jay Jay" as he leafed through a dozen or so envelopes lying on his desk. "Oh yes here they are, been ready a while, why haven't you collected them before?"

"Sorry" I said, as if it was my fault. And then came a moment that made everything an anti-climax.

"Here you are then" he gruffed.

"Thank you I said" reaching out for them

"They're perfectly clear you know," his voice seemed a little less gruff "well done my friend" he said as if I had been personally responsible. He gave me a large twinkling eyed grin, and I picked up the envelope as if I had won the lottery, said "Thank you" yet again, rushed out to the car and said to Polly – "Hey….Guess what?"

I almost ran into Winterlands.

"Hi girls" I said to the ladies of reception,"or as they say in good old España, *hola chicas*". I beamed, waiting for them to be impressed. I could see them fighting the laughter. "Be so kind as to give this small picture of my bones to Dr. D, I do believe he is waiting for them" one of the girls stretched out her hand and took hold of the envelope "do be careful" I said, "I'm rather ticklish"

"Oh go a sit down" she said "if anybody wants you they will call for you" but she was laughing. I sat down and hummed a little chorus of "*The Road To Mandalay*"

Jo came along. "Hello Mr. Jay, did you have a good time in Tenerife? I bet you're glad to be back in a changeable climate"

"I'm getting acclimatized" I said, there is nothing quite like February in Maidstone"

"No" she agreed, "***nothing*** is quite like it" and then, without changing pace, Dr. Draper said "would you both like to come in."

We both went in.

"Well Mr. Jay" rather more formal than Mr. B's booming "WELL NOW BASIL" it made one feel that he had a sombre voice for a sombre moment.

He had a sheath of what appeared to be X-Ray photographs on his desk, and alongside them a single sheet of paper on which he was drumming his long, beautifully manicured fingers. "I don't go in for the 'Good News, Bad News' approach" he continued, but, there is, I am afraid a little of both." I did the old scrunching up the toes into the bottom of the shoe trick, suddenly realizing that my Mr.

Gruff had only had the result of the bone scan. That was obviously the *good news,* the *bad,* would obviously be that the MRI scan showed the cancer growing all over the place. I forced myself to answer calmly. "Oh, a little of both…I see" I said no more, I saw no reason to make it easy for me.

"Your PSA has risen to 0.7, and that is definitely *not* good, it means that it has increased more than seven fold in less than three months. That in turn indicates that there is something cancerous left, and that it is growing quite rapidly" He actually smiled, how can you deliver a statement like that and then actually smile as if he had just told you that you had won this months Glamorous Grandmother competition. His smile grew broader, and just when I thought he had to be a sadist in pin stripes he said.

"I told you there was good news, and there is, the best. The cancer has not spread to either the bones or the surrounding tissue. The bone scan is clear" he sort of wagged a finger at me "but you knew that didn't you" I nodded

"Yes", I said "Dr. Gruff told me"

"Dr. who….."

"No Dr Gruff"

"Oh you must have seen Dr. Simpson" He didn't pursue the subject; instead he said: "What we have is a bit of rogue cell tissue that Mr. B unfortunately left behind" YIPEEEE. The smiles were forgiven; in fact I gave him a grin that made the traffic lights change in Maidstone High Street.

"So where do we go from here?" we said in stereo, me as a question and he as a direction. I deferred to him and leaned back in my chair.

"Prostate cancer" he began "feeds off testosterone" I nodded sagely. "What we must do therefore is depress the testosterone" he was sure as hell beginning to depress me. "How do we do it?" He continued. He doesn't know, I thought, but before I could develop the thought, he continued "the answer is, of course, obvious" Of course it is, I said to myself, a sharp knife and a stiff upper lip, and 'Bob's your uncle…or maybe your aunt. "We have to feed you the female hormone oestrogen" I look aghast, he smiled and explained. "The male and female hormones don't get on you see, and the female hormone will immediately get the upper hand and depress the male hormone". It was a long explanation and he paused for breath, I took the pause as an opportunity to enlighten him about a couple of things.

"Hormones" I said, "are obviously like real people in real life. The female takes the upper hand and the male gets depressed." He nearly smiled, but his eyes said, *please try to be serious.* I tried to be serious. "Sorry for my flippancy" I said, "but you have just given me a bit of cloud nine news", and I'm trying to make the best of it before you bring me back to terra corridor" He actually did smile this time.

"OK", he said briskly, "let me tell you what I propose." He then began to tell me what he proposed. "First I want to get that PSA back down as low as possible…hopefully back to 0.1" I nodded, he didn't. "The oestrogen will do that" he said, "but, he paused, and then said slowly, "unfortunately it will do other things as well"

"Oh" I said "side effects"

"Side effects" he said, "exactly so" and then continued briskly, "but let's come back to that in a moment, first the programme." He opened up his diary. "It is now February 14th"

"Valentines Day" I said

"Valentines Day" he agreed

"Valentines Day" added Polly who hadn't contributed much to the conversation so far, no doubt savouring the prospect of us both being girls together.

"I want you to take oestrogen, orally for four months.

31

If you start on", he flipped a page of his diary, "the 21st February, that will take you through to the 21st June."

"What about the side eff.....", he cut me off, kindly, but firmly.

"let's get the programme sorted out first" he said, "and then I will tell you exactly what you can expect." A soft voice said

"OK"...... It was mine.

"Where were we?" He studied his diary, "providing your PSA is down, at the end of that session, I want to immediately start you on four weeks of daily radiation therapy. That will take you up to 21st July."

"My 64th birthday" I said in a small voice, looking at Polly and remembering Paul McCartney's 1960's song *'will you still need me, will you still feed me WHEN I'M SIXTY FOUR'*. Being unable to read my mind, Dr. D simply said, "No it's not, your birthdays is the 28th'" he was looking at my record card. Polly nodded in agreement; I simply looked sheepish and said

"Oh yes....sorry" Dr. D had that *'poor old man'* look in his eyes, and I would swear that he started speaking a little slower.

"I will then want to leave it a full month
before we carry out a few tests,"

"Does he take sugar?" I wanted to say, remembering a half forgotten programme about how people tend to treat *'poor old men' as* if they weren't there. Then Dr. D flashed me a big grin, and I realized that he had only been extracting the Michael. His sense of humour was battling its way past his professional exterior. He carried on at normal pace, "and then by the end of August we will know exactly where we are."

"That sounds good to me," I said, but now can we....."

"Run through the side effects" he finished for me. "Of

course we can." I waited for the list of feeling nauseous, feeling tired, feeling depressed etc and was confident that I could deal with them all. He began.

"The most obvious *'side'* affect for a man, is usually the noticeable growth of the breast tissue. Remember, that for four months we will be giving you the female hormone oestrogen" He waited for my nod to show that I was keeping up". I nodded to show that I was keeping up.

"Now, hormones affect the make up of the body. Tell me, what is the major physical difference between men and women", I knew this one.

"Women have long hair and like to paint their toenails"

"Yes" he said "and"

"Women have high pitched voices and make shopping lists"

"Yes, and something more fundamental". Aha, I was now on his wave length.

"Women" I said with a knowing air, "have sticky out jumpers"

"Absolutely" he applauded me, "and they don't buy them in M&S"

He put on his serious face, "After ten days or so", he said *in a poor you, sort of voice,* you will experience a tenderness in the nipple area, and then, gradually you will notice that your breasts are becoming larger" I was speechless, "You will also experience hot flushes, you will almost certainly put on a little weight, you may become depressed, your skin may begin to irritate". Not as much as your explanation I thought. "And you may find that your libido, your sex drive, will perceptibly lessen as the testosterone is overcome by the oestrogen"

"Oh my God" I thought, "I am going to become a *middle aged woman*". "After the four months treatment is completed", he continued, and provided it is not necessary to repeat it, your natural hormone balance will re-assert itself and those characteristics *might* disappear." Sadly, he placed more emphasis on the *might* than I *hoped* was strictly necessary. Was I speechless, I was beside myself? Laughing boy hadn't finished yet. "And then", he said to both of me, "we will start the radiation therapy, and that produces a different set of side affects which could include, skin irritation, tiredness, even lethargy, nausea, hair-loss around the area to be treated, and skin burn"

"It sounds like a walk in the park" I said. He smiled.

"You are taking it very well" he said.

"I have already found two tremendous pluses" I replied

"Oh"

"Firstly, the testosterone is suppressed so there is less danger of my becoming infatuated by my own sticky out jumper"

"Good point" he said

"And secondly, if the worse comes to the worse, I can always make a few bob as a Dolly Parton look alike"

"You will need to put a paper bag over your head" he said, and at that point I considered the consultation over, and it nearly was.

"Basil" he said, and that was the very first time he had called me by my first name in this consultation, "what is about to happen is not an easy ride, but when anyone can face what will be a pretty unpleasant six months and retain their sense of humour, they have won the biggest battle of all" I said nothing, and it was a good job because he hadn't finished. "Just bear this one thought in mind. The cancer has not spread, we are dealing with some localized cell tissue which was left behind after the operation, it is growing very rapidly, but we can eliminate it before it spreads, and we will" It seemed to me that at this stage we should all have clasped hands and said *'All for one, and one for all, D'tanyan'*.

Polly, ever practical, asked the question I had overlooked.

"Dr. Draper" she said, "do you want us to stay in England now?"

"Absolutely not" said Dr. D, you can take your medication as easily in the sun as in the rain. You just go back and have a restful winter until......" he looked at his diary, "the end of May, because then I will need you to come back and have a series of scans during which we will give you a tattoo to pin point where the radiation treatment will be aimed". He stood up, so did we. He thrust out his hand. We thrust ours back in a *we are all in this together* sort of way. He grasped mine, and I grasped his. He opened the door for us. We walked through it. "Goodbye" he said

"Thank you" I said. The door closed and he was gone. I was reminded of the old saying, *one door closes and another one slams in you face.*

It was clearly time for me to face my Tigers.

Chapter 6

A TIME OF GROWTH
(FEBRUARY – JUNE 2007)

There are two things I want to make clear. The first is that Dr. D was *wrong* about the effect of depressed testosterone on my libido…YIPPPEEEE so Ladies, don't stop elbowing yourselves to the head of the queue. The second is that a sticky out jumper on a woman is very fetching. A sticky out jumper on a man poses more than one question. BUT, I must here praise the Daily mail for putting things in perspective. I name them happily in the belief that 'product placement' as the best marketeers call it, may well result in them offering me immense wealth in return for the serialization rights of this book. That wonderfully generous newspaper ran a double page spread that proves beyond doubt that, 'sticky out' male jumpers are far more common than you would suppose. In fact, it ran a series of articles *and pictures,* of the male predominant boob, called….wait for it *a moob.* There were 'swimming trunks only' clad photos of Tony Blair, Michael Winner, Jack Nicholson, Simon Cowell and others, all sporting, perhaps no more than a 34 A. cup, but sporting it for all that. I suddenly felt that my *MOOBS* would be in good company, as indeed were my *hot flushes*. But I get ahead of myself; easily done when your Moobs lead the way. Let me chronologicalise that unusual four months.

A couple of days after the consultation I had to return to the hospital to collect four months supply of boob enhancer. I was told to discontinue my regular simvastatin (for lowering my cholesterol) whilst the oestrogen was doing its work. I accepted the fact that my cholesterol level might well rise in time with my breast diameter (or should it be circumference). One thing did intrigue me, and that was, that wanting to be well informed and in control, to some extent, of my final body shape, I had spent an hour or two on the internet and had discovered a cosmetic clinical site that specialised in,.....here it comes.....*male breast reduction*. Now, on the site there were a number of photographs of men of a variety of ages who had a need for the procedure. Some offered the smallest of firmly thrusted mounds, whilst others confirmed the old adage that, in the fullness of time everything heads south. Humpty dumps that, from the neck down to the waist, could have *graced* the upper torso of many a lady of uncertain age *(obviously my profound apologies to any Graces who may read this book).*

Now, there was one thing that intrigued me, and that was why the hairiest chest still offered a quite bald moob. It was true, some torsos looked like Sherwood Forest, with Ben Nevis (or should it be Bernice Nevis) poking above the tree tops. Other torsos had fine hair like gentle waters of the South Seas lapping a desert isle, whilst from the centre thrust twin peaks that were as smooth as a baby's bottom, or the virgin sands of Robinson Crusoe land. Somehow, that looked more unacceptable than having hairy breasts – in any event, I was now fore-warned and simply had to discuss the matter with my Tigers.

After several serious talks with my Tigers, we reached a sort of understanding – and I will share those discussions with you a little later.

But first, armed with my four months supply of oestrogen, in the form of a tablet called Bicalutamide, Polly and I set of for the winter sun once more.

Dr. D was right about so many things, but wrong about others. The sensitive nipples. He had that right, and in spades. For the first week there were no visible signs of appearing moobs, nor physical discomfort. And then, towards the end of one particularly warm day, I became very conscious of my silk shirt rubbing uncomfortably on my chest. I looked in the bathroom mirror and just for the moment thought that someone must have pushed a couple of button mushrooms down my shirt front when I wasn't looking. I opened my shirt. Oh dear! Oh dear! Oh dear! What on earth could have got me into that state of excitement? Suffering from the vaguest feeling of embarrassment *(we were entertaining friends at the time)* I changed into a black cotton shirt which seemed to successfully hide my phantom excitement. I rejoined the party explaining that the white silk shirt was a little warm, and I thought a cotton one would be cooler. There ensued animated discussion which roughly translated appeared to be saying….How stupid are you….you're hot so you put on a BLACK shirt, everybody knows that WHITE repels heat and BLACK attracts it, that's why cricket teams wear whites. I nodded my agreement, but at that stage felt quite unable to tell them about my mushroom stalks. As the days passed I watched my burgeoning breasts with the horror of a pre-pubescent school girl. In time, I became less embarrassed, but before that happy time, worse was to come.

So, I had the tingly nipples. One up to Dr. D. The libido however was functioning one hundred and ten per cent. One up to Basil J. You are probably dying to know if the four tons of Viagra, taken since the last book had done the job....die on my friends, all *(well nearly all)* will be revealed a little nearer the end of this book. First I want to talk about '*hot flushes*'. Lord help us and save us, I always thought '*hot flushes*' were a female fantasy rather akin to the '*vapours*' suffered by the hoop dressed, long-bloomered ladies of Victorian England. I can tell you now.....a fantasy they are not, from imagination they do not come, a neurosis, not at all. They are unpleasant, they are uncomfortable, and they are embarrassing. Some of my favourite blouses have been quite ruined. Do I not like hot flushes?

As time passed by, I began to identify myself with the girls, I brought a little electric fan so I could sit outside and blow the hot air *(hot air and Basil, it has been said, have never been strangers)*. We girls would sip our pina colados and talk about grandchildren and shopping trips, about handbags and leotards, about crochet and cooking. No we would not, I held tight to my macho belief that the heat came from the sun, and only serious work-outs made you sweat. But I still carried my little battery fan, and changed my blouse two or three times a day.

Was the oestrogen putting me in touch with my feminine side? Of course it wasn't. Was it making me weepy or broody? Absolutely not. Was it making me want to clean, cook, and iron? No chance. Was it making me want to talk a lot, shop a lot, rest a lot, sun bathe a lot, read a lot, or even choc a lot? Not a lot. Was I getting debilitating nocturnal headaches, concerns about messing up my hair or my make-up, worries about creasing my dress, an unconscious desire to slap the hand that caressed me, a desire to use unpopular literary phrases like *"Not here"* or *"There's a time and a place?"* On all of these questions I tested myself and found myself not wanting. Well, perhaps wanting, but not getting, if you know what I mean. On reflection I decided that after four months on serious oestrogen, my libido was intact, my performance was unmarred, and my machoness was

unimpaired, and my boobs were about 36D cup. I had put on about 2 stone in weight and ten years in feminine intuition. I had, as Mr. B once told me, been to the brink and looked over. I could now recognize dust from several inches, I knew instinctively when the curtains needed washing, and I actually started to worry about the missing sock. I had had the irritating skin, the moments of depression, the total loss of any sense of direction, the complete inability to read a map, the natural tendency to turn the wrong way when coming out of a hotel bedroom, the inexplicable urge to read Mills and Boon and watch 'weepies' on the television. In short, I feared I was mutating. Through March and through April I was terrified in Tenerife. In May I was adjusting in Ashford. In June I was Ecstatic in Eire, and so my spring and summer drifted by. I was put in mind of that wonderful novel *The Prime of Miss Jean Brodie.* We had surely seen the prime of Basilina Jay. My oestrogen intake stopped on June 21st, and gradually I stopped feeling my feminine side, and began to pay attention to the male side I intended to take back to Tenerife.

But first, the ordeal of the Radio Therapy. I had had my tattoo, and they knew exactly where to aim, so now nothing separated me from four weeks of daily doses of radiation, and a host of experiences that were going to both lighten and darken my life for the month of July, because, on the 21st day of July, just seven days before my 64th birthday, I was to be dealt a hand that would have made a poker player cry….

and it had nothing to do with my health. Certainly on that day I was confronted with a group of people who felt, they DID need me, and WOULD feed me, even *though* I was *sixty-four.* BUT I WASN'T GOING TO LIKE IT.

CHAPTER 7

A MOTLEY CREW
(JUNE – JULY 2007)

My first radiation appointment was at 11 am on June 21st. I arrived in good time, signed in on a sheet of paper that listed my every appointment for the next four weeks, and which the receptionist highlighted to show that you had turned up for that particular day's treatment. My sheet showed a full page of entries and just one broad yellow band. I longed for that day when it would be reversed, but that was still four weeks away.

Having signed in I put on my blue slippers, as provided, and, finding a seat that looked out over a splendid courtyard, I settled down to read, the most up to date copy of the Readers Digest that was sitting on a small table. Wasn't it terrible about that Titanic? I was about to get into the detail when I felt somebody touch my arm.

"Hello" he said, "first time?"

"Good Morning" I replied, "yes, how did you know?"

"Your slippers ain't not got no holes in them," he said,

clearly proud of his double negative. I looked around at half a dozen or more blue clad tootsies. Sure enough, they were in various stages of collapse, some barely holding together. I looked at mine. They were absolutely pristine.

"Ahh" I said, "I see what you mean".

"Names Cyril" he said, "done 4 weeks, just two to go"

"Basil" I rejoined, "first day of four weeks"

"It's not so bad" he said, "better than the old breast manure"

"Oh" I said, "you had the hormone therapy too"

"Been there, done it, got the T shirt" he said. I cringed; I had obviously sat next to the last of the original thinkers, but I tried not to be double negative. Please spare me, I prayed, the joke about how you make a hormone. He spared me the joke about how you make a hormone. Miraculously, whilst I was saying my silent please don'ts, he was getting quite seriously verbal. I caught up with him.

"Bloody stuff made me put on a barrel of lard, and my boobs would look well on Sabrina" Sabrina, I thought, that puts an age tag on you. "It's made me fat, a bit, and frankly, I don't think I'm going to get rid of it easily." Fat-a-bit and frankly. What a perfect moniker for my new friend Cyril. Cyril out, ***Fat-a-bit and-Frankly*** in. I let him ramble on whilst I started my new game of giving appropriate epitepths to the group who were probably going to join me on this radiation trip of discovery. Over in the corner, his right ankle over his left knee, pulling at the sole of his pretty blue slipper was a thin, bald man, looking as if he didn't know what day it was. ***Bald-But-Bewildered*** I decided to name him; it occurred to me that he had clearly not been exposed to the boob enhancer. Then it further occurred to me that, of course, only those of us who had had prostate cancer would probably have needed oestrogen, and only those of us who had taken a course of oestrogen would have expanded their horizons, at the same time as they broadened their breasts. I reflected that there were other cancers that needed treatment by radiation. I had to break of my thoughts processes to throw a quick,

"Oh you are so right" to ***Fat-a-Bit-and-Frankly.*** Like a good meal for a hungry man, or a gallon of diesel for a JCB, this injection of interest seemed to stoke him up enough to launch into another session of his unintended soliloquy.

To pass the time, and shut out the steady stream of chatter, I decided to list the possible cancers requiring radiation starting from the top of the head. I could feel the poetry coursing through my poetical nerve ends.

There's cancer of the Cranium and maybe of the Brainium,
Although it gets your goat, there is cancer of the throat,
But you need never fear that you'll get cancer of the ear,
Nor do I suppose there is cancer of the Nose.
Even if you're young you could get cancer of the tongue
But the mouth or teeth, my friend, will never bring your end.
I really quite forget if there is cancer of the neck,
And if I may be bolder is there cancer of the shoulder
But the one we all know best is cancer of the breast,
For a gal, but for the rest perhaps its cancer of the chest.
If your hubby don't feel well 'ee, may have cancer of the belly
The thighs, the knees, the calves, don't get cancer, not by halves
Nor do ankles, feet or toes, but that's just the way it goes.
I had a pal called Roger, thought he'd cancer of the Todger
That's wrong, but it isn't mystical to get cancer of the tisticle.
I'm being quite absurd. That's the worst thing that I've heard.
But even if you're thin, you can get cancer of the skin
And the Bladder and the Bowel is a cancer that's most foul.
But the one I do not rate, is the 'my now gone' Prostate.

My attention was suddenly arrested by a tap on my arm and a voice echoing loudly clear across the room
"Basil Jay".

Fat-a-Bit-and-Frankly had stopped talking and was tapping me on the arm. "That must be you Basil". I looked up, the young man who had tattooed me was standing at the door of what I later found out was the radiation room. "That's young Gerry," said ***Fat-a-Bit-and-Frankly,*** he's a *nice boy,* know what I mean, nudge nudge, wink, wink" ***Fat-a-Bit-and-Frankly*** was obviously a Monty Python fan, *nudge nudge, winks as good as a nod to a blind man,* I flashed him a smile, said,

"Nice talking to you Cyril, see you again no doubt" and pointed my pristine blue slippers towards Gerry.

"You'll see me tomorrer" ***Fat-a-Bit-and-Frankly*** called out to me, we all seem to come at the same time every day. "Nice talking to you" I waved, and as I turned my attention to the radiation room door and Gerry, I realized that I was actually looking forward to seeing him tomorrer.

"He's a new boy" I heard somebody say, "Just look at his slippers"

"Hello Basil" said Gerry "I remember you, you live in Tenerife don't you?"

"Hello" I strained to see his name badge, I couldn't quite recall his name from my last visit, and I felt that it was a bit risky to take the unsupported word of ***Fat-a-Bit-and-Frankly.***

"Hello.......Josh" I said, managing to read the badge and noting that it bore no resemblance to Gerry whatsoever.

"Not Josh, its Gerry" he said, I couldn't find my coat so just grabbed the first one I came to"

"Oh", I said, "Gerry, I'm sorry, I should have remembered"

"Good job I didn't get Priscilla's coat" he chuckled, "That's got sticky-out bits" I laughed politely, wondering whether he was poking fun, but I don't think he was. "walk this way" he said, I resisted the temptation to the old joke, if I could walk that way you could call me Gladys, and I walked that way.

In the room which was around a long curved wall obviously designed to keep the killer rays aimed at the one place they were supposed to be aimed, there was a low couch and a huge barrel like contraption. "Just take you trousers off, lie down and make yourself comfortable" he said. I checked his name badge just to make sure. A young lady in her early twenties joined us.

"Hello" she looked at her clip board "Basil" she finished "I'm Kate"

"Hello Kate" I said. She put what felt like a small wooden ramp under my legs and said "I have to just slip you pants down, but when I've seen what I want to see I'll pop a blanket over you to spare your blushes. What an earth I wondered, did I have that she would want to see? Before I could develop the thought Gerry chipped in.

"She means your tattoo Basil; we have to line the machine up on three sides with the tattoo we put there so that we make certain that we hit the spot."

"Fine" I said, "I don't know whether I was relieved or disappointed."

"Now said Kate, just let yourself sink into the couch, don't help me or try to move at all." She then proceeded to tug me first one way and then the other, lifting me one moment, pushing down on me the next, whilst Gerry called out strings of meaningless numbers. At last he said.

"That's fine." He repeated the numbers to Kate, and Kate repeated them back to him. Obviously cross checking. Then,

"All lined up Basil" said Kate, "the machine will now pivot first on your right side, then on your left side, and then from above and give you three, timed bursts. The machine makes lots of odd clicking noises, but don't worry about them, it knows what its doing. And then with a cheery wave they both left the room.

The lights in the ceiling dimmed, and, no doubt controlled by Kate or Gerry from a remote room, the machine began its work. The first time, I listened to every click and buzz. I watched the flashing lights... flash; I watched the ceiling lights which went on and off....go on and off. I tuned into the power noise as the machine rotated, and tried to remember each sequence. I was sure that as day followed day I would be able to predict each revolution. Each bleep, each click and each buzz.

I worked out that, whilst the machine was assimilating the information from the computer, the ceiling lights came on. As soon as it gave a strange little 'I'm ready now, Burp' the ceiling lights went off. A series of clicks like a car engine cooling followed, and then a prolonged buzz. I found that when pointing at my right side I could count up to one hundred in the way I, long ago, taught my children to count off the seconds.

One Mississippi, two Mississippi, three Mississippi etc. etc.

Then the ceiling lights would come back on again. The scanner would revolve and settle on my, now, ample middle, the machine would Burp, the lights would go out, the clicks would begin, and then the buzz.

One Mississippi, two Mississippi, three Mississippi and so on.

This time the machine seemed to stop at a count of about seventy. On came the lights, around went the scanner to focus on my left side, the friendly burp, off went the lights, click click clickerty click click. Then the buzzing.

One Mississippi, two Mississippi, three Mississippi. Usually up to one hundred again. And then back would come Gerry and Kate, or Rakeem and Sophia, of Josh and Joanne. Or whoever happened to be on duty. All done Basil, you can pull up your knickers and strides, OR its OK to put your pants and trousers back on, OR time to make yourself respectable again. They all had their own little way of making you feel at ease. They really were a splendid set of young people.

As I left the radiation room after that first visit, **Fat-a-Bit-and-Frankly,** *was* standing at the entrance, obviously next up.

"Enjoyed our chat Basil" he said, he winked at me *"Nice boy* is Gerry....see you tomorrer then." And he was gone, and, as I have already said, strangely enough I was actually looking forward to seeing him *tomorrer.*

As time went on I got less interested in the burps and the clicks, in the buzzes and the whirrs, and just lay sometimes adding to my poetic cancer location saga, but more often re-living conversations I had had with my various new brothers in arms, to say nothing of breasts and prostates. The deterioration of the interest in the progress of treatment seemed strangely linked to the deterioration of the blue slippers as day followed day. I was told I would feel lethargic, and frankly, wanting to please, I really tried, but somehow I just couldn't be bothered. I was told my hair would fall out....It didn't. I was told my skin would suffer from irritation. It did. I was told I would feel nauseas some of the time. I did. But I was not alone, and whilst my formula for getting through was observing my compatriots, my compatriots all had there own way of getting through the waiting and the treatment. As day followed dreary day, I got to talk to many of them, and in fact, after **Fat-A-Bit-And-Frankly,** took to naming them after either their open comments, or sometimes their oft repeat ones. Take **Mr. They're-A-Nice-Lot-In-Here-Ya-Know,** He had sat down next to me on about my fourth visit. Judging by his slippers he must have been at least a five weeker. "Wotcher", he said bringing his lips right up to my ear "Their-a-nice-lot-in-here-ya-know"

"They do seem very nice" I replied

"Especially young Gerry"

"Yes I've met Gerry" I answered

"And Kate"

"and Kate" I said

"and Rakeem" he looked at me expectantly

"I'v haven't met Rakeem" I said

"No you wont have done" he replied "he's on holiday, but Their-a-nice-lot-in-here-ya-know" I just nodded, but that didn't stop him from going through the whole list. Josie, Jan,

Mandy, Josh, Sophie, Michael, Nick. At first I just used to nod, but eventually I would just nod-off, to be usually awoken by

"Come on Basil, it's your turn."

Take Joke-**A-Day-Jeffrey.** He started each greeting with "Hey hey Basil, this'll make you laugh" We knew it would corny, we knew he would probably forget the punch-line, but **Joke-A-Day-Jeffrey** was a tonic. I remember the first joke he told me.

"They are very professional in here" he said, "incidentally, do you know the difference between a professional and an amateur"

"Go on" I said

"Well" continued *Joke-a-Day'* "A professional is a man who can do his job , even when he dosen't feel like it, and an amateur is a man who can't do his job, even when he does feel like it"

If I thought that was the worst I would be subjected to, I was soon to be seen the error of my hopes when he followed up with "Basil, this'll make you laugh.

Young man gets his fountain pen stuck in the photocopier when he was trying to sort out a paper jam. He went to his boss. "Sorry sir, I seem to have got my pen jammed in the

photocopier." His boss tells him to phone the engineers and in the meantime put a notice on the copier saying it was out of order. Boss goes to lunch. When he returns, all the office staff are having convulsions. He walks over to the copier to see this notice. **Joke-a-day** produced a dog-eared piece of car with the punch line written on it.

> ### OUT OF ORDER.
> ### PEN IS STUCK IN WORKS.

"Hey Hey Basil, that made you laugh", pretty appropriate for most of us eh! eh! eh! And strangely enough, it usually did make me laugh.

There was **Mr. Nice but Nervous,** Every day he would sidle up to somebody and say, "I say, I'm not interrupting you am I, before embarking on a harrowing tale of parking his car, or dead heading the flowers, or some other disastrous domestic chore which he was nervously expected to tackle. **Mr. Hail-Fellow-Well-Met**, was your typical larger than life character whose voice boomed across the waiting room and up and down the corridors as he would call out. "Hey there Basil, how are doing then, eh….eh." A simple nod was usually the only response he needed because he always had other fish to fry. **Mr. Hirsute-But-Heroic**, had the biggest beard I have ever seen, black, bushy and definitely grown in memory Walter Scott's famous quotation **"Oh what a tangled web we weave"**. It has to be said that **Hirsute-But-Heroic's** beard was as tangled a web as you are ever likely to see, and must have housed at least a dozen nesting House Martins and the odd Cuckoo. His whole demeanor was one of Victorian Tragedian. And then, last and most definitely least, **Mr. I-Thought-I-Only-Had-A-Cyst'**.

As the weeks progress, I was fortunate in that my side effects were not as dramatic as had been the front effects of the hormone treatment. However, I did experience days of total lethargy, some skin irritation, occasional nausea and general un-wellness. And one day my leg fell off. No it didn't I just made that up. Actually, I pinched that off of *Joke-A-Day-Jeffrey*

"Hey Hey Basil, This'll make ya laugh, man has a blinding headache, he'd had it for weeks and tried everything, but it wouldn't't go away. In despair he went into a new chemist shop. "You've got to help me, he said, I'm going mad with this headache, I've tried everything and it just gets worse". The chemist offered him, Aspirin, then Paracetamol, "I've tried it", said the man, "can't you just make something up" The chemist offered him Codeine, then Ibuprofen and the man just yelled "I've tried everything, can't you make something up". The Chemist walked into his laboratory, and was back in a few minutes with a small bottle on which he was writing. Standing at the counter he said, conversationally, "Frank Sinatra was in here today", the man was enthralled. Was he really he said in awe. "Nope", said the chemist, "I just made it up.........
here's your aspirin"

Hey Hey Basil, I bet you liked that one."

And so the days rolled one into another, my little menagerie of comrades waxed and waned as old ones finished their courses of treatment and new ones took their places. I was gradually becoming one of the old hands, one of the elder statesmen.

I was just two days from the end of my treatment when an event occurred that almost changed my life, an event that I would never in a thousand years have thought I would experience. An event that even rebounded on Polly. An event that sets you apart from your fellow man.

At 8.21am on the morning of July 21ˢᵗ 2007 I was arrested on suspicion of money laundering..............and so was Polly

CHAPTER 8

WE'VE GOT THE BUILDERS IN (JULY 2007)

What happened to us both at 8.21 on July 21st 2007 was so un-expected, so absurd, so horrific, so TV black comedy, so life experience enhancing *(I'll explain that later)* that 24 hours after the event I recorded everything that had happened so that I would never forget. One day I might write a book, I will probably call it *"a day in the life of a criminal"*. In the account that follows the names have been changed to protect the guilty, who, it would appear in the eyes of the law, are every man-jack of us.

The sun was forcing its way through the bedroom curtains of our west facing bedroom, which considering that it was in the back garden at the time was no mean feat. There was not exactly a lot of noise outside, but one sensed, in a curious way, movement. I slightly lifted the curtains and peered out. A car had parked right across our driveway. Silly Sod, I muttered, how the hell does he think I am going to get out – at that point it would not have occurred to me in my wildest dreams that he did not want me to get out. We live on a small private road with just four properties. Ours is at the entrance, and in fact the title of our home includes the private road that serves them. I noticed that another car had parked diagonally across the end of our small road in such a way that *no-one* could leave the close. Still no pennies dropped. "There are a couple of guys outside," I said to Polly "who are either drunk or stupid, and at this time of the morning they must be stupid. They have blocked us all in, I am going to go out and have a word before they vanish". I let the curtain drop quite unaware that several more cars had now pulled up and the forces were gathering. I pulled on a shirt and some trousers, a pair of shoes without socks, and walked from the bedroom *(we sleep on the ground floor)* through the hall, into the outer lobby, and was about to open the door when there was a loud hammering thereon which must have raised a hundred heads in the nearby church graveyard. I turned the key, and then the handle, but before I could even begin to pull the door open it was shouldered wide, banging loudly against the door jam. A man wearing a scruffy blue waistcoat and brandishing, what appeared to be his credit card, walked straight into me pushing me backwards whilst yelling at several hundred decibels above that that was needed

"YOU ARE BASIL JAY"

"Yes…who ar….."

"CUSTOMS AND EXCISE…..YOU ARE UNDER ARREST." He might just have well been speaking a foreign language for all the sense he was making. People were filing past the two of us, I didn't count them but I later discovered there were eight of them including two women. The women immediately grabbed Polly, who had followed me into the hallway, one on each elbow and propelled her back into the bedroom. Two of the men then grabbed me in similar fashion and almost frog-marched me into the lounge. I noticed they both had guns, albeit holstered, at their belts, and the scruffy blue jackets were 'flack jackets', some with POLICE, and others with CUSTOMS AND EXCISE emblazoned across the back. They had obviously heard of Basil Jay the criminal desperado.

"Have you got any weapons in the house?" yelled the top man, at the top of his voice. I later learned that his name was, and for that matter probably still is, Chris Hilton. We live just fifteen minutes from the Euro Star terminal, but they could hear his voice in Calais.

"Of course I haven't" I said not believing that such a question could be asked of me. Basil Jay, friend to everyone, enemy to none, of whom a speeding fine is a major event that I haven't experienced since 1986.

"Have you got any money in the house?" the volume had not softened one iota.

"Only what's in my wallet or my wife's handbag", I said in a small, totally disbelieving that this was happening, sort of voice.

"Have you got any drugs in the house?"

"Of course I bloody haven't" I snapped back, I was still horror stricken that this was happening to me, but I was also beginning to get pissed off, and matched him decibel for decibel "**and who the hell are you and what are you doing in my house at 8.00 o'clock in the morning**" I bared my tooth at him - I felt like rushing into the bathroom, grabbing the full set, baring them all and really scaring him. I'm joking of course............I don't keep them in the bathroom.

"You just keep quiet, and do what I tell you when I tell you to do it"

"I'm f***d if I will"** Now everybody who knows me knows that SWEAR I do not, so you get the measure of how they were getting to me.

"I'm 64, I have never done anything criminally wrong in my life, I have cancer, I have radiation treatment every morning, INCLUDING today in just 40 minutes time, you burst into my house, you say nothing more than CUSTOMS AND EXCISE, you frog march me into the lounge and my wife into the bedroom, and I am f****d if I am going to say another word to you until you give me an explanation." I was panting from the exertion "and it better be f***ing good." I was now shouting louder than he had. It had a strange affect; he simply looked at his colleague and said,

"John, read him his rights." A tall good looking lad in his mid thirties, dressed in a smart dark suit and highly polished shoes – no flack jacket in sight, turned to me.

"Basil Jay, we are arresting you on suspicion of money laundering, you don't have to say anything, but anything you do say etc...etc....etc....." He was talking calmly, and the words just washed over me, meaningless, but, at the same time full of meaning. This, whatever it was, was really happening. How the hell could such a mistake have occurred? Was it April 1st, were they members of the village Parish Council dressed up. My mind was blank, and so must have been my stare, because, John, obviously playing the good cop, and having finished his premier performance said.

"Are you OK Basil?"

"Can I sit down?" I said, moving towards the settee.

"You will do nothing unless I tell you that you can do it" yelled hardman Chris, **"John, check the cushions"** good cop John, lifted the scatter cushions and then the seat cushions and looked under them. Hardman Chris grabbed them off him and flung them to one side. Having satisfied himself that I did not have a couple of sub machine guns hidden there he yelled **"Sit down and sit still"**

I sat down and my body sat still but my mouth moved quite a lot.

"Look" I said in a conciliatory fashion, trying desperately to remember scenes from Z cars or Fabian of the Yard. "I absolutely do not know what this is about, what I do know is that the only money that I have ever laundered is the odd five pound note I have left in a shirt pocket before it went into the washing machine." I waited for the laugh, it didn't happen. "Now then" I continued, "in time you will find out what I have just told you is true, and what is happening now is a mistake on the same level as believing in Santa Claus. Whether or not you believe it now is irrelevant. BUT, and this is a very big BUT….I most certainly have cancer, I really have had major, life threatening surgery, I am most definitely undergoing a properly structured series of treatments. I have one, now" I looked at my watch, in just twenty minutes time. You know, and I know, that if you deny me that treatment **AND I DIE**, *(I thought it would do no harm to be a bit, alright then a lot, melodramatic)* your careers end… today….in this room." I paused, for effect. "Particularly when you all discover how absurd this arrest is. Now then, do you not think that you better go and make a phone call?" He went and made a phone call, whilst I reflected on the fact that he was younger than my youngest son. He didn't go without wanting the last word, and stalked through the lounge door *(which fortunately was open at the time)* looking over his shoulder as he said loudly **"Keep an eye on him John"** He was gone about five minutes. He walked back into the lounge looking as if someone had kicked him in the balls, I hoped they had. He still spoke at top volume.

"Listen to me….we know who you are, and we know what you've done" he winked at nice cop John **"We've got Mark Southerby and he's told us everything"**. Praise the Lord and pass the ammunition, I thought, they really do act like this, they really are absolute bloody arseholes, AND they are making me swear even in my head. I couldn't ignore him.

"Look, I said, that is the third lie you have told me" I waited for him to say something like

"No it isn't - I've only told you two", but it was obviously his turn with the brain cell, because he just stared at me.

"*I* know it's a lie and what's more important *you* know it's a lie. There will come a time, believe me, when you will discover that everything I tell you has been the truth, because, unlike you. *I* don't tell lies." I wanted to add *because I'm a golfer,* but he wouldn't have understood, I did go on "So for your own sake, don't tell me too many more lies because I will make *bloody* sure that when this is all over, each and every one will come back and bite you on the backside." I felt good after that little speech, but was soon made to realise that I had been a dammed fool to think I could take them on. Mr. Macho Man ignored me.

"You'll do exactly what we tell you now, and if you co-operate we will take you to the hospital for your treatment before we take you to the cells to lock you up" Obviously his boss had told him to make bloody sure that I got my treatment at the hospital and that *he* got the paperwork in triplicate. I raised my eyebrows but said nothing. **"Now, we have a search warrant and we are going to tear this place apart. Make it easy for yourself and us. Have you got a safety deposit box?"**

"No"

"And you _say_ you have no money in the house" before I could answer a voice called down the stairs.

"Chris there's a safe up here in the cupboard on the landing" Macho Man Chris yanked me up by the elbow, **"Get up those stairs now" he yelled. "You said you had no safe in the house"**

"You asked" I answered in my best Chairman of the Board voice, "if I had a safety deposit box. I have not. To the educated world a safety deposit box is a box in a remote location, such as a bank, or a specialist security facility what your man has located is just a domestic safe and………." I just stopped talking and raised my eyes heavenwards, the fact was, I was now getting pretty much pissed off by, not only the facts that these hooligans were stamping around my home, but by the attitude of Macho Man Chris. " I was trying my best to be quietly patronizing but he cut in with….

"Keep it closed…..just give me the key" we were now on the landing where the cupboard and the safe were located. A man was kneeling at floor level taking out the books and papers which were alongside and in front of the safe and theoretically hiding it.

"I don't have a key" I said, now, *knowing that I was absolutely innocent of anything,* beginning to enjoy myself……. or was I just kidding myself.

"Are you telling me that you have a safe but you don't have a key to it?"

"Yes" I said

"So you never open it, is that it" he said, with a sneer.

"I open it most days" I said smiling.

"Chris" from the man on the floor

"Leave it Alex, I'll deal with this" then to me "So what's in this safe *that you don't have a key to?"* He had decided to swap volume for sarcasm, and it is difficult to be sarcastic at 300 decibels.

"Well" I said, "My wife's jewellery, a couple of nice watches, our passports. I think a couple of cheque books and….." I paused….*"about three million dollars".*

"THREE MILLION DOLLARS" I swear he nearly

wet himself. "Is that the truth", he hissed, a statement, NOT a question.

"I told you" I said "I don't lie.....but" I added, "they are Zimbabwean dollars"

"Zimbabwean" he said, quieter now, and then suddenly **"So, *you don't have a key.*"** He had decided he *could* do sarcasm at 300 decibels.

"Chris", insistent now from on the floor, where he had knelt beside his oppo. Alex. "There won't be a key, it's a combination lock. Poor, Macho Man Chris, I almost felt sorry for him, but I hardened my heart. His antics bore a striking resemblance to Peter Sellers in his craziest Inspector Clouseau moments.

"Why didn't you tell me?" he yelled

"You didn't exactly give me much chance" I said

"Do you know the combination?"

"Of course I do, it's the only way I can open the safe".

"What is it?"

"I'm not prepared to tell you"

"*You're what!*"

"I'm not prepared to tell you...BUT, I will open the safe for you"

I got the impression that I was winning, but as the day progressed I realized that antagonizing Macho Man was not a clever move. For the moment however I was actually enjoying myself – or am I still kidding myself again.

"You are saying that you will not co-operate"

"On the contrary, I am saying I will open the safe for you, what I am not prepared to do is give you the combination, because if I did that I would never feel my personal possessions were safe in the safe again"

"Chris", it was good cop John, "Let him open the safe." He let me open the safe. Macho Man was straight down on his knees. He pulled out Polly's jewell boxes and rifled through them. I have a passion for watches, and I had four in the safe, including a 30 year old Cartier a Vacheron Constantin, a Krug Baumer, and a limited edition (10 of 100) German watch which made the *'Best Watches of the World'* top hundred in 1997. Four watches worth collectively well in excess of 'just a little', and not far short of 'quite a lot'…but they might just as well have been a Timex, A Mickey Mouse, A Gerald Ratner 'crap' special, and a Lookeee Lookeee man's most obvious ……..philistine. But, I knew what he was looking for, he was looking for **THREE MILLION DOLLARS,** and he had not yet worked out that that much *real* cash would not fit into a domestic safe, 14 inches, by 10 inches, by 9inches.

"Where's the cash?" he yelled. I leaned over his shoulder and pulled out six or seven crumpled bank notes in a rubber band. He missed that action. He was too busy working himself up into an orgasm. *"Where's this Three million dollars?"* This time more quietly, and with a sneer. I held out the notes in front of him. Without thinking he reached forward and took them from me.

"Well" **he** said, ignoring his small handful and building himself up to a crescendo.

"You're holding them" I answered, "they are Zimbabwean," I couldn't resist adding; "like I told you" I took the notes from his hand, and counted them back to him. One note was for 1,000,000 dollars.

"One Million" I said, there were two for 500,000 dollars each, I counted them into his hand "one million five hundred thousand, two million" I said. The remaining two were each for 250,000 dollars, I put both into his hand together, "and another half million makes two million, five hundred thousand." I smiled at him, "Sorry," I said, I could have sworn I had *three million*" I paused and then said" Perhaps I've been robbed, there have been some unsavoury characters about recently" One thing I must say was always in Macho Man's favour, that was that he never rose to the bait, never once. As usual he ignored my comment and scowled.

"How much is this worth?"

"Well, I said, when we were on holiday in Zimbabwe last year, the taxi from airport to the Victoria Falls hotel cost us 750,000 dollars, and two gin and tonics in the Hotel bar were 500,000 dollars. So I would guess that the total value is between ten and twelve pounds sterling." Macho Man was NOT amused. Was he NOT amused? But I suddenly realized what a bloody fool I had been to make him look an idiot in front of his men.

I tried to recover the situation. "My hospital appointment is at nine thirty, I said, it is now twenty past, can I at least telephone the radiation department and tell them I will be late"

"I'll do it" he said, incredibly his voice had returned to usual volume.

"I would be grateful if I could do it" I said

"That will be OK Mr. Jay" this from John, "That's OK isn't it Chris, we don't want to make the hospital visit more difficult?"

"I'll get the number" said Chris, "you can speak to them"

"I really appreciate this" I said, and gave him the number. He dialed on his mobile

"Is that Maidstone Hospital.....Radiation ward please?"

"Oncology Department" I whispered. But they put him through anyway.

"Are you expecting Mr. Basil Jay for treatment this morning?" he said. They obviously said yes. "This is the police," he said, grinning at me "we have him in custody,

61

but he wants a word with you". He handed me his mobile. Quick as a flash I said loudly, and solely for the benefit of Rose, who I believed was duty receptionist this day, and who I had been seeing virtually every day for the past month. "Chris, you really are a card, but one day somebody may take you seriously, and then you'll get into trouble"

He scowled at me for reversing the position. "Hi Rose" I said, "It's Basil Jay, I've got a bit held up and will be a bit late…is that OK? How long…." I looked at Macho Man. He took the phone from me.

"He'll get there when he gets there he said…..we have a lot to do here". He'd got his own back……. in spades.

"We have a lot to do here," he repeated, and it seemed that they had, but little of it was going to affect Polly or I. As I handed the phone back to Macho Man I had looked over the bannisters to see Polly, still with an escort on each arm, being ushered out of the door from the inner hall.

"Polly" I called out

"You can't talk to her" yelled Macho Man "She's got her own questions to answer"

"Where is she going?" I asked, noting that they were now already out of the front door.

"Dover Cop Shop" said Macho Man.

"Dover" I said incredulously, "Why the hell Dover?"

"Can't risk you both in the same place, can we" he sniggered.

"You must think us pretty dangerous, if you think it necessary to interview us 50 miles apart", I said, at last realizing that we could both just be deep in the doo doo, and were about to be locked in up in a couple of remote cells.

Eventually, he led me out of the house. As we reached the front door John put a hand on Macho Man's shoulder and whispered in his ear. Macho Man nodded, and said.

"Before we leave John has something to say to you. John produced his notebook, and holding it in front of my eyes said…I need you sign my book to confirm the notes I have made…please read them" I read them, but didn't really take them in. They said in effect that they had knocked at my door at 8.21 on the morning of July 21st and ascertained that I was Basil Jay. That they had then 'escorted me', into the lounge where they had read me my rights. That I had opened the safe for them voluntarily, and that I had no complaints about the way I had been treated. Polly was now long gone and was probably being beaten by police batons on the soles of her feet until she confessed to knowingly putting that five pound note into the washing machine. I assumed she had been asked to do the same. Although Macho Man had shouted a lot, in essence John had recorded the happenings more or less accurately, and as I was anxious to get to the hospital. I signed.

As we passed Polly's car in the drive, *(my car, which had almost 5 euros in small coins in the ashtray, was, thankfully, in Tenerife)* Macho Man called over his shoulder to Alex, who was clearly his favourite and most faithful lap dog.

"Alex" he said, "Gimme the car keys" I had watched Alex take the keys off the key hook as we left the house.

"Here Chris" he said, handing them over. Macho Man gave them to me.

"Open the car he said" I opened the car. There was a small, shirt pocket size note book on the passenger seat. I picked it up and put it in my shirt pocket.

"What's that?" he shouted, shattering windows in about three surrounding cul de sacs.

"It's a note book, I usually carry one because I'm a writer" OK, a little massaging of the truth wasn't going to hurt. He grabbed it from me and opened it at random.

"What's that?" he said, pointing at a page.

"Its writing", I replied frostily "you may not recognize it because it's joined up." John gave me a frown which suggested *'take it easy, it's not worth scoring points'.* Macho Man ignored the jibe. He took it from me and threw it to his bag man.

"Bag it Alex" he said. As he led me to his car two more cars drew up in the close and a few more bodies fell out. He put his hand on top of my head and pushed me down and into the back seat *(yes they really do do that).* He followed me in. John climbed in the driving seat and started the engine. As we pulled out of the close I looked through the back window. People were swarming everywhere, over the car, the garden shed, even the cloches outside the kitchen window.

"Where's the Hospital?" asked John. I told him. Apart from me giving directions and John asking "Now where?", the drive was almost silent. Macho Man, now and again threw in a comment that was obviously meant to scare the life out of me. They never did. There I go, kidding myself again.

"We have all the bank statements you know" He sneered, I said nothing. "I just asked you a question" he said

"No you didn't", I answered, "you made a statement, and statements do not require answers". There seemed little point in winding him up and telling him it was a 'bank statement'.

"We have an affidavit from the bank manager" I ignored it

"You're in a lot of trouble" this time I did answer

"I cannot imagine that I am in any trouble at all, and I have the advantage over you. I know the truth, and the truth is that I have done absolutely NOTHING wrong, and therefore do not need to defend myself." I paused, "and right now I am more worried about the fact that I have cancer, that you are taking me to hospital for radiation treatment that has been going on every day for almost four weeks." I turned and looked at him. "Let me tell you this. When you ask me specific questions I will answer them, what is more I will answer them truthfully." I could not resist adding "I suspect that you are more a stranger to the truth than I am." I took a final gamble. "I don't want to offend you, but, I am not going to speak again until after my hospital treatment, until after we have arrived at the police station, and until after *you have bloody well told me what this is all about*"

I turned and faced front. So did he, but, for the rest of the journey none of us said a word beyond the occasional "turn left here" or "right at the lights." When we arrived at the hospital car park, something happened that really put things in perspective. Now then, remember, we are in a perfectly ordinary unmarked saloon car. The hospital car park was, as always, very busy and as we drove very slowly looking for a parking space, a lady tapped on the driver's window. John let it down

"Young man" she said, "I am just going, my car is that one" she pointed to a blue Fiat. "Look" she said "there is about two hours left on my ticket, you may as well have it" she handed it to John, who said

"That's kind, thank you very much". After we parked, Macho Man said,

"Hey that's a result John, you can get the ticket cost back on expenses" I looked at him and raised my eyebrows. He didn't pursue the subject. He knew, that I now knew, that not only did he tell lies, he was dishonest as well. Why was I not surprised.

They got me out of the car. Hand on top of head. They stood one each side of me with a hand on my elbow. They just fell short of carrying me as they ushered me through the entrance. At least I wasn't in handcuffs. What happened next was the stuff of mini-nightmares for an innocent man. Rose was at reception,

"Oh Basil," she said "you've brought your friends with you", but the look in her eye made it obvious that she knew that *friends* they were not. She put a line through my name with a sad smile….tomorrow, I would have to explain. We went through to the waiting room. ***Bald but Bewildered,*** started to say hello, but seeing two unsmiling faces shoulder to shoulder on me like bodyguards, he sized up the situation, thought better of it and just nodded. ***Joke a Day Jeffrey*** didn't have a joke; he just looked at his shoes. There were half a dozen of my regular 'buddies' there, and, except for the odd nod of recognition, they had all found the most amazingly interesting article in their copy of Readers Digest or House and Home. We sat apart from the others in three connected chairs. Me in the middle, Macho Man on my right, and John on my left. John eased me forward and leaned behind me to whisper in Macho Man's ear. "When he goes in for treatment" said Macho Man "I know how hot you must be" Macho Man called a passing porter over, and saying, "keep an eye on him" to John, got up and, taking him gently by the arm whilst chatting to him, walked him around the corner.

"What's all that about?" I asked John, who really wasn't a bad sort.

"I expect he's just checking where all the exits are in case you do a runner" he smiled, realizing that that particular scenario was pretty unlikely. John was also half wrong. Macho Man had been to see Gerry, who happened to be on duty with Kate, to ask that they see me next. They did. When we got to the curved wall entrance to the radiation room Macho Man started walking towards it.

"You can't go in there, it's dangerous" said Gerry. "Are there any doors out of that room" asked Macho Man.

"No" said Gerry

"We'll see" said Macho Man" who had obviously read Dale Carnegie's book on how to win friends and influence people. He stomped off. He came back and said to me "OK, you can go in" I raised my eyebrows to Gerry who looked rather embarrassed. Once in the room Kate joined us. You must remember that I had got to know these two lovely people pretty well over the past four weeks, and they me.

"What an earth is all that about?" said Kate

"I wish, I knew" I answered "Hopefully all will soon be revealed

"It's obviously more than a parking offence" said Gerry

"As far as I'm concerned, it's no offence at all I said"

"Well good luck" said Kate "we better get started. You know the drill" I took my trousers off and lowered my Y fronts whilst Kate pushed me and prodded me into position. They left the room. I was quite oblivious to the clicks and buzzes; my mind was fixed on one thing. What could all this be about? Kate and Gerry came back and I got dressed.

"Bye Basil" they said together "I hope we will see you tomorrow" said Kate.

"So do I" I answered, and walked out of the room. Macho Man was waiting for me and as we walked back into the waiting room John hurried up carrying a green plastic bag.

"Better son?" said Macho Man

"Much" answered John

"Never wear the vest myself" carried on Macho Man, "much prefer the flack jacket it's easier to get out of". The problem had been solved.

We got back to the car. I notice he did not offer his unused car park ticket to any of the waiting motorists. "Where's Maidstone Police Station?" asked John

"Turn left at the entrance, then left at the second lights" I said, then straight on, about 2 miles, into the town centre". It crossed my mind that I could keep them driving around for hours, but I had long since decided that I wanted to get this sorted out sooner rather than later, and a magical mystery tour would not improve Macho Man's temper any.

Now, I am not a fool, and although I knew I had done nothing wrong, I also knew that when you are Chairman of a company that incorporates off shore tax structures, you may unwittingly have provided services for someone who has. At last count my old company from which, although now retired, I was Life Chairman, had incorporated and, in many cases managed, well over 5,000 companies over the previous few years. Some clients I knew well, some I knew vaguely, but, particularly since my retirement in 1999, most I did not. What I did know was that we were licensed by the Financial Services Commission in Gibraltar, and we did everything, always, by the book. Our due diligence was second to none. All I could do was be patient and let Macho Man give me a little information. I sat back and in due course we were let into the underground car park of the police station that had a door leading straight up a flight of concrete stairs to the cells.

I will not bore you with the hour I spent, with my two new *best friends* in the Holding Cell whilst they waited to process me and find me a cell of my own. Eventually I was taken up to the duty officer who took my details, and details of the alleged crime, as provided by Macho Man. He checked that I was in good health. I told him that I had cancer that I had come straight from the hospital that I was just coming to the end of a course of four weeks of daily radiation treatment, that I had just finished four months of hormonal therapy, that I had a radical prostatectomy just 20 months early. He listened, wrote it down, said "Fine, now empty your pockets. All of them." I did, he gave me a receipt for about sixty pounds in notes, a few coins, and a handkerchief. Then said "Now stand on that line for a photograph" I did as I was bid. The duty sergeant then turned to Macho Man "Cell 3 at the end of the corridor. The duty jailor will take him. Then when you are ready we will free up an interview room for you." Macho Man's answer made me want to tell duty sergeant about the car parking ticket. But I didn't.

"Fine" responded Macho Man, "But first things first, where's the canteen? I am starving and we need a good breakfast before me start work." The duty jailer arrived rattling his keys.

"Basil Jay, cell 3" he said

"Rightho" said the duty jailer" and to me "Down the end of the corridor and wait by the gate." I went, I waited. He came up behind me with a second officer who opened the gate. I walked through the gate, and to my surprise, on my left was an open shower where a man in his fifties was having a good soap. There was no door, not even a curtain. We got to the end of the corridor. Cell 3 was on the left.

"Take off your belt and your shoes" said the jailer. I did. I'll have your pen as well" he said pointing to my Caron d'Arche gold pen which I had stupidly grabbed and put in my shirt pocket as we left the house, and which had somehow been overlooked by the duty sergeant, together with my Cancer, Radiation and Chemo-Therapy. The door was opened; I was ushered in and left to my own devices. The cell was about six by six with a moulded concrete bench and a moulded concrete toilet. No seat. No privacy. In fact so much did it **not** have privacy that a CCTV camera which I would swear was trained from the corner of the cell directly on to the loo. I sat on the bench, and, whilst imagining Macho Man and John tucking into bacon and eggs, and poor Polly experiencing much the same as me in Dover, I began to assemble my thoughts.

It was 11.30 before they came for me. It had been three hours since they had hammered on my door and turned my little world upside down. The duty jailer and his pal unlocked the door of my cell and walked me, between them, back along the corridor, past the now empty shower, through the locked gates and into an interview room. I was bursting for a wee, a problem that had become more acute since my surgery.

"Sit down…there" said Macho Man pointing at a chair on the opposite side of the desk at which he and John were comfortably sitting, a plastic coffee cup by their elbows…

"I would like to use the loo first" I said

"Why didn't you use the one in your cell?" he scowled

"because," I answered, "in my 64 years I have never once had a pee on camera, and I do not intend to start now"

"worried about your dignity?" sneered Macho Man, **"crims don't deserve dignity"**

"Crims" I queried

"Criminals" helped out John

"I thought," I said, "that in England people were *innocent* until proved guilty – which means by definition, it is not possible to be a criminal, until you have been found guilty of a crime and collected a criminal record" I looked at them both. "So, which loo can I use? there's one just outside this door" I added. The door was still open and they both looked at out. A sign above the door said **W.C. – NOT FOR THE USE OF PRISONERS** Macho Man immediately saw his chance. **"You may not be a criminal….yet"** he said, "but you are certainly a prisoner".

"You will either let me use that loo, or I pee on the floor right here" I said, bursting and no longer caring. They opened the door to the WC.

I felt I was winning small victories, but the **big** game still lay ahead. Macho Man read me a prepared statement about my rights, he offered me a lawyer, taking care to let me know that I could easily wait for three hours or so for a duty lawyer to be found, and that time would be spent locked in my cell. He tried hard, unsuccessfully, to hide the fact that he too would have to wait three hours, and so delay his return to the seedy sordid streets that he obviously loved to frequent in London's East End.

I declined a lawyer, for my sake rather than his. He then spent ten minutes trying to work out how to use a tape recorder, and explaining to me what it was for. A further minute or two was devoted to confirming who I was, reminding me of my rights, of having me agree that I had been offered a lawyer and declined, and was being treated well. Finally, when all of this was over, praise be, John asked me if I would like a cup of coffee. I said yes, and shortly afterwards, when I was presented with a cardboard beaker of dirty grey liquid, wished I hadn't. As the day progressed I must have had half a dozen more.

Eventually, we were all set, and Macho Man had his stage.

"Do you know what a carousel is?"

"Yes". He seemed taken aback.

"Yes".

"Yes". Have you ever been involved in a carousel?

"I wouldn't say involved, but just a month ago I took my grandson to the Palace of Versailles, and they had a funfair with one of those *really* old fashioned carousels, you know the kind, with the candy striped poles and the grinning, high step…….."

"What are you talking about?" he said

"A carousel" I said

"A carousel" he said "is a VAT fraud"

"No it's not", I said, it's a Round-A-Bout, a Merry-Go-Round, a popular addition to every village fair since the Middle Ages."

"A carousel is a VAT fraud" he repeated

"Well," I said, "what an earth would I know about that?"

"So you **say** you're not familiar with a VAT Carousel" he said

"I've never heard of one" I said

"Are you a director of a company called BASIS MANAGEMENT Ltd?" He asked

"I don't know" I answered honestly

"You are telling me you don't know if you are the director of a company"

"That is not what I said", I said, "I am the director of many companies, what I don't know is whether I am a director of a company called BASIS MANAGEMENT Ltd"

"You expect me to believe that?"

"I really don't care" I said, the truth is the truth, and the truth cannot be altered. He made some notes, and then spent a minute or two reading them, no doubt hoping to unsettle me.

"How many companies are you a director of?" he spat

"I don't know" I replied, but with one phone call I would be able to tell you.

"So", he sneered **"you want to phone a friend – where do you think you are?…..on *who wants to be a***

millionaire" He preened himself and waited for laughter. He got none from me, and simply a polite, *'good one boss'* sort of a chuckle from John. I ignored him

"I asked you a question" he said

"It was rhetorical" I answered "rhetorical questions don't presume an answer",

"Suppose I told you that we have *proof* that NOT ONLY are you a director of BASIS MANAGEMENT LIMITED, BUT SO IS YOUR WIFE, and NOT ONLY are you the BANK SIGNATORY on the account BUT SO IS YOUR WIFE...WHAT WOULD YOU SAY?"

"I would say that both I and my wife are directors of BASIS MANAGEMENT Ltd and that we are both bank signatories"

"AHHH" he said "so you admit it"

"You promised not to lie to me again" I said, and you have just said that you have *proof,* so I am content to accept what you say as a fact"

"Oh, it's a fact alright" he gloated

"I would also say, that we would hold those positions in a nominee capacity, that my old company would hold beneficial owner declaration and indemnities in each case, that they would hold, on file, FULL and COMPLETE due diligence on the beneficial owners, and that our nominee status would be registered in the country of jurisdiction of the company in question" I leaned back in my chair. So did he with his mouth sagging open. Eventually he spoke to me

"Would you like to explain all of that?" he said

"First" I said, "bearing in mind that I want to resolve whatever is going on here" I paused and looked from one to the other, "can I ask you both a question or three" they stayed silent, so I asked counting them off on my fingers.

"one.......do you know what I used to do for a living

before I retired? Two…..do you know when I retired? Three…..do you know what a CSP is?…………And four….. are you familiar with the term voluntary disclosure?"

"Why don't you tell us" snarled Macho Man, determined to prove he wasn't a buffoon.

"OK, hopefully this will explain, what for you is pretty inexplicable. I first retired at the end of 1989 and went to live in the Isle of Man in1990. "How old were you?" broke in John, the quiet one.

"Shut up John" said Macho Man, "let him speak". I ignored Macho Man.

"I was forty-eight" I said. "Anyway, for three years I did nothing except play golf and write. But it wasn't enough and I became very bored, so, in 1992 I bought the controlling interest in a company called Crouch Waterfall Ltd. It was a Jersey Company, a CSP" – seeing their blank looks, I expanded. "CSP stands for Corporate Service Provider, which, in simple terms meant that the Crouch Waterfall Ltd incorporated Limited Companies, and set up foundations and trusts all over the world. Part of the 'Corporate Service' functions would be providing, Registered Offices, Nominee Directors, Company Secretaries, Bank Signatories, and Nominee Shareholders. All of these functions were, and still are, provided in a nominee capacity. The Beneficial Owner held a legal Deed, or Declaration of Trust provided by the nominees affirming that all of the offices were filled in a nominee capacity, that the nominees had no legal or beneficial interest in the company and that all executive officer operations would only be carried out on the written instruction of the beneficial owner" I paused, to let them take it in. "Any questions?" I asked, Macho Man just said

"Carry on, *we* will tell *you* if we have any questions". Determined to keep control, and frankly, he was doing so badly that I really didn't blame him.

"OK, having acquired control of the company in 1992, I ran it until 1999, when I semi-retired though retaining full ownership until 2001 when I transferred 50% to my, now, CEO. Since then I have worked only in a consultancy capacity although, I am Life Chairman of the Company. This was one of the very few conditions of the transfer. The company, incidentally now has offices in England, Gibraltar, Tenerife and Bulgaria."

"Tell me about BASIS MANAGEMENT Ltd"

"I can't"

"You expect me to believe that?"

"I've already told you, I really don't care whether you do or you don't, but the truth will always be the truth"

"How can you be a director, owner, and bank signatory of a company and not know?"

"Since I acquired my company I have been director, shareholder and bank signatory for many hundreds of companies that my CSP has incorporated. It may come as a surprise to you but I remember the names of only a handful"

"Do you know the name Mark Southerby?"

"Yes I do"

Ahh, you do, where do you know him from?"

"I don't know him"

"You have just said you did"

"No I did not; you asked me if I knew the *name* Mark Southerby and I agreed I did"

"You are telling me that you know the name, but not the man"

"I am, yes"

"Where do you the name from?"

"Earlier today, you told me that a certain Mark Southerby had told you everything"

"Now you are being a smart ass"

"Listen, I told you in the hospital that everything I tell you today or any day will be the truth. If I may say so, you phrase questions very carelessly; you seem NOT to know the difference between a statement or a question, or whether a question is interrogative or rhetorical. I will continue to answer *the questions you ask*, truthfully and completely. If you want different answers, I suggest you give a little thought to the way you ask the questions." Good cop John was frowning a warning at me again. Macho Man said

"Are you trying to be clever?"

"No, I am trying to ensure that there are no misunderstandings. I am beginning to see the problem you have, how my name has become entangled, and, believe it or not, I have always, all my life been on the side of the good guys, which, I *think*, puts US on the same side. So can I suggest that you get a little less confrontational, and, if you do, I well may be able to help you"

"Big speech" he was clearly still not prepared to concede "but you haven't convinced me yet"

"OK, let me tell you about Voluntary Disclosure. All of what I am about to tell you is capable of being verified at the highest police and customs level on the Isle of Man. Now can I ask you again, do you understand what is meant by Voluntary Disclosure?"

"Explain what *you* understand by it" Macho Man was clearly NOT prepared to admit he did not know.

"It is not a question of what I *understand* about Voluntary Disclosure, it is a question of what I *know* about it, because, I may not have written the manual, but I certainly wrote a chapter or two during a more than a decade on the Isle of Man." I paused and looked at them both, and, from the vacant looks on their faces, realised for the first time that I had obviously become fluent in Swahili. "OK," I continued, beginning to feel sorry for them having thought they were dealing with a simple company matter, and now finding themselves entangled in an offshore world that they had clearly never had a moments briefing on. "Let me give you a couple of working examples of VD". I paused to let him catch up and to ensure that he understood the acronym was for helping the authorities and not a sexually transmitted disease. "Right, in the early 1990's we incorporated and provided the full corporate package – that, as I have explained, includes, **nominee** Directors, Company Secretary, Shareholders, Registered Office, **and** bank signatories. The company was called Montevideo Developments Ltd. This company was soon showing a very high cash flow, and, with all the paperwork in place we managed the company, purely from a statutory books point of view." I paused, they nodded. "After about a year, a returned postal package arrived at our office *(as the Registered Office of Montevidea)* with *ADDRESSEE UNKNOWN* stamped on the envelope. We opened the envelope to find its source, and were confronted with a package of pornography of the very worst kind. I immediately called the vice squad and set up a meeting. I passed over the package and told the investigating officers I intended to resign all positions immediately. They confirmed that that was my right, but that it would greatly assist them if I would keep everyone in place and carry on as *'business as usual'*. That way they would be able to monitor all activity, including intercepting post. In the event it took almost two years, but one day at Ronaldsway Airport, I was waiting for a flight to Liverpool when The DI in charge of the case came and stood by my chair and said.

"Hi. Basil, you can resign now. We got the bastards, 20 arrests, about 500 grands worth of porn, and a whole printing operation. Thanks for your help." I stopped talking and stared at each in turn willing them to take in what I had just told them. I then continued.

"Voluntary Disclosure meant that we were NOT mentioned at any time either pre or post arrest. Our efforts were important and appreciated, and more particularly were carried out in a jurisdiction that understood what 'Nominees' really were." Macho Man and John were both silent. "Between 1992 and 1999 my company was instrumental in bringing to an end five major scams. Including Montevideo, a Prescription Drugs scam which had netted the perpetrators almost 2 million pounds in just 13 months, and a cheque washing operation, which began in the United Sates and ended up in the Isle of Man." I then gave Macho Man the names of three law enforcement officers, one in the vice squad and two in HMRC that I had worked with on the island, and told him to check it out. He suspended the interview and told me that he needed to consult his boss. I was led back to the cell where I spent another two and half hours before the Jailer came and took me back to the interview room. I could not believe it, it was if the previous interview had not happened.

"I have here a copy of an affidavit from Mr. Neil Bainbridge, the Managing Director of Crellin's bank in the Isle of Man" he started. **"It was sworn less than thirty minutes ago in front of the"** he put his glasses on and stared at the paper in his hand **"Chief Deeper….."**

"Chief Deemster", I corrected him, "It means senior judge" He went to carry on, but I held up my hand. He stopped and looked expectantly.

"Do you recall", I said "that, at approximately 9am this morning…some hours ago, you told me that Mark Southerby had told you everything…*and* that you held a affidavit from my bank manager, yet now you tell me the affidavit was only signed thirty minutes ago" I sat there waiting for him to give some explanation. He just carried on as if I had not spoken.

"and it says that you were the beneficial owner of
BASIS MANAGEMENT Ltd" **What do you have to say
about that?**"

"May I see the affidavit" I said. He handed it to me. I
read it.

"Do you understand" I asked, "the difference between
a shareholder and a beneficial owner?"

**"What I understand, smart arse, is that Mr.
Bainbridge tells us, under oath that you were the
beneficial owner of BASIS MANAGEMENT LIMITED."**
I handed the affidavit to him.

"Show me," I said patiently, "exactly where it says that".
He took the paper, reluctantly, I thought, and started to read
it. He read it again, and then flipped over to an attachment.
Jubilantly he stabbed his finger on a section of a form.

"There" he said **"Right there"** I took the affidavit back
and read out loud.

"Number of shares issued..........TWO.

"Name of Shareholder/s ....BASIL JAY" I paused
and looked at him. Then I tapped the affidavit with my
finger. "I can't see the words BENEFICIAL OWNER" I
said. "Perhaps I am missing something"

"Mr. Bainbridge clearly says that according to bank
records ALL of the shares in BASIS MANAGEMENT Ltd
are held by Basil Jay"

"I agree" I said. "What Mr. Bainbridge does NOT say
is that Basil Jay is the BENEFICIAL OWNER OF Basis
Management Ltd....Do you know why he does not say
that?" No response, so I continued **"Because** I am NOT the
Beneficial Owner.....let me make the phone call I asked
for several hours ago and I will tell you exactly WHO the
beneficial owner is ....accept, I said, that *I won't,* because
under my company's confidentiality agreements we can only
pass on such information if given JUST CAUSE. So far

you have given me nothing except a pain in the arse." I was losing my cool now **"Perhaps I should talk to someone with an IQ greater than that of a cockroach"** Of course, I regretted it immediately, but luckily, having an IQ lower than a cockroach he didn't notice, he just called the jailer and had me taken back to my cell.

About 2.30 I received a call in my cell from the duty inspector who, apparently by law, had to make sure I was OK, had neither hung myself nor stuck my head down the toilet, and had everything I wanted …. except of course, my freedom.

I lied. I told him I had no complaints.

"Have you had anything to eat?" he said

"No" I said

"Are your hungry?" he said

"No" I said

"Have you had something to drink?" he said

"Only coffee" I said

"Would you like something else?" he said

"Yes please" I said.

"What?" he said

"A Gin and Tonic would be nice" I said

"I'm sorry" he said "alcohol is not possible"

"Oh" I said

"Would you like something to read?" he said

"What is there?" I asked

"Various magazines" he said, and then before I could answer "I will tell the jailer to bring you something"

"If you have no complaints" he said "I will log this call at 2.33 and will speak to you again when required"

"Goodbye" I said. He didn't answer and the phone went dead. However within two or three minutes the jailer had brought me a copy of a magazine called 'Boys Stuff, a great disappointment, it was all about fancy gadgets, and a copy of country life. Pictures of wide open spaces. Yes, I am sure you get the irony. Having little or no interest in **that** kind of 'boys stuff', I leaned back against the moulded concrete of my bench. I closed my eyes and let my mind wander over the day's events.

*Suddenly the door was slammed back against its hinges and Macho Man came in. For some reason he was now in uniform and carrying a pair of handcuffs and a truncheon. "Stand up **NOW**" he yelled. I stood up, and he forced my arm up my back, and frog-marched, me to the concrete toilet, and stuffed my head down it whilst pulling the chain. "**ADMIT IT**" he yelled. Suddenly I felt a kerfuffle behind me and the weight was lifted from my neck. I pulled my head out of the loo and turned around. The lovely Nita had Macho Man in a headlock, and was pushing an elephant sized syringe into his, now exposed buttock.*

I heard the door open, I opened my eyes. I was sitting on the bench with a copy of *'Boys Stuff'* on my lap. I must have momentarily dozed off. What a good job all of this nonsense was not getting to me

"Come on my friend" said the jailer, who hadn't been all bad, "they're ready for you again."

"I know who you are" said macho man

"So do I" I said,

"I've decided to tell you all about the carousel"

"What you mean" I said, "is that during your coffee break you have phoned your boss and he has told you to tell me all about the carousel in case I can help you" He ignored the jibe.

"It is normally worked with either mobile phones or computer chips" he started. "There is a company; we will call it A Limited. A Limited sells a consignment of mobile phones; let us say to B Limited for £500,000 **PLUS VAT of £87,500.** B Limited then sells them to C Limited for £700,000 **PLUS VAT OF £122,500.** C Limited sells to D Limited etc. etc. and so the carousel is formed. There may be a dozen companies in it. Each one CLAIMS BACK the VAT, and when the final company has supposedly bought the phones, it puts itself into liquidation. And although hundreds of thousands has been paid out in reclaimed VAT, no company ever coughs up to HMRC. In the case in which BASIS MANAGEMENT is involved, the total VAT repaid on numerous consignments of mobile phones is in excess of FIFTY MILLION POUNDS. Your company rec….."

I interrupted him

"For the benefit of the tape" I said, Basis Management Limited IS NOT my company"

"Do you deny that you were a director?"

"I have already told you, I don't know if I was a director, but I would be no more surprised to find that my company had provided a corporate nominee package for the beneficial owner of Basis Management, than I would for any one of around 5,000 companies you could name going back over the past fifteen years"

"You expect me to believe that"

"I have already told you", I said, a little tersely, "I really don't care if you believe it or not, because the truth will out…. eventually. The company files are immaculate and would provide the fullest possible details of the beneficial owner/s of any company we manage"

"So you will give me those details?"

"I won't, but the office will, providing always", I continued "that you obtain a court order"

"Why would you want a court order?" said Macho Man

"The company has, what a duty of care, a fiduciary

duty to its clients. That duty implies full and complete confidentiality, BUT, if there is sufficient evidence of wrong doing, then the company is absolutely on the side of the good guys, a court order is the one certain way of ensuring that there is such compelling evidence of illegal activity." I was warming to the theme "too often over many years, you have used absurdly draconian powers to complete little fishing expeditions that should never have been started in the first place, you then walk away with not so much as an apology, leaving innocent people to put their lives together again."

"Is this your signature?" he said, as if I had not even spoken. He handed me a sheet of paper that I immediately recognized as a photocopy of one of the company's standard international bank transfer requests.

"Possibly," I said, "although it could be a signature stamp"

"So you admit that you transferred the sum of" he paused and squinted over his half moon glasses at the sheet of paper "£750,000 pounds sterling to" another squint "this bank here" he tapped the paper so forcefully with his index finger that it tore, "a bank," he leaned forward conspiratorially "not connected to the United Kingdom."

"The bank", I said "is Barclays , one of the *big four* High Street Banks, whom I am sure would be most upset to learn that they are not connected to the United Kingdom. The branch of Barclays" I added, is Gibraltar, which whilst being a sovereign state, is a British protectorate, and, I am sure, that there is not a Gibraltarian who would not be offended by your assumption"

"Where did the money come from?" he said

"I have no idea", I said, but you appear to have a sheaf of bank statements in front of you, you have a dated transfer request, or what is left of it in your hand, and if you try really hard I expect you could bring the two facts together and find out where the money came from" John squirmed in his seat, but frankly I didn't care any more. Macho Man was a joke, and as I already knew, a dishonest, lying, joke at that. He had a habit of ignoring me. He ignored me now, but at least he did rifle through the bank statements, and, after peering at one for a few seconds, jabbed at an entry and then handed the statement to me.

"Right he said, there it is in black and white, £750,000 with the narrative BENSONS CLIENTS ACCOUNT, beside it, now what do you say?" I was tempted to express surprise that he knew a word as long as *narrative*. Instead I took the statement and barely glanced at it, because, of course, I recognized the name.

"Have you checked on the source of these funds?" I asked.

"Hardly a need for that" he said, "when you are going to tell us what we need to know" I was having fun because two items above the £750,000 item, I had found one for £1700 which was very telling.

"OK", I said, I will tell you exactly where the money came from". He leaned back in his chair with a smug look on his face. "Before I do," I said "can I ask you a straight forward question?"

"What?"

"Do you not think it would have been sensible to trace any items you were concerned about to their source, and even exercise a little bit of common sense, before storming in and arresting, not only me, but my wife, for money laundering?"

"Go on"

"BENSONS" I said, are just about the largest firm of commercial lawyers in the North West of England. Head office in Liverpool. Their 'clients account' is in one of the major clearing banks. I don't know which one, so for the purpose of this discussion"

"Interview" he interrupted

"Alright, iinterview, Let us say it is with Nat West. OK, so your hypothesis is that, I Basil Jay, and my wife set up an account, in the name of Basis Management Ltd. We give the bank our full names, and a copy of our passports. We give them two utility bills as proof of our private address. We then sit back and prepare to collect a part of a fifty million pound VAT swindle, and hide it in an secret offshore account, except, of course, the secret offshore account is hardly a secret, because it is in another branch of Barclays in Gibraltar. No paper trail there then". I looked at them. They both sat there po faced, so I continue. "But we haven't finished yet; we then manage to persuade a very large, and eminently reputable, firm of lawyers to pass three quarters of a million pounds through their client's bank account at say Nat West, in Liverpool." I stopped talking and looked from one po face to the other. "Does it", I asked, "seem plausible so far?" Macho Man however was nothing if not single minded *(always assuming he had a mind at all)*

"So what was that money for?"

"Taking into consideration the source, I would guess it was for some commercial property deal…why on earth don't you ask Bensons?"

"Oh we will, don't you worry about that, we will". There was no point in responding so I didn't; instead I directed them to the other item on the bank statement.

"I've already said that my office will not disclose the beneficial owners name without a court order. You have presumably obtained a court order to acquire these bank statements, and I have to tell you that even from glancing at just one of them, a route to the beneficial owner is obvious."

"Oh" he was interested now. "To who does the account belong then?"

"To whom" I said, I hate bad English "what is the entry two above your magic £750,000?" He looked

"£1700" he said

"There is a narrative showing who the money was ppayable to" I said. He squinted at the paper over the top of his reading glasses.

"St Richard's School" he said. "Why would you transfer money to St Richard's School?"

"Obviously because my office was instructed to, and the instruction could only come from……" I paused so that Macho Man could wind up the brain cell. He was too slow.

"The beneficial owner" interceded John

"So what is obvious then?" said Macho Man.

"The point is" I said slowly, "that payment was probably school fees. If you go to St Richard's School and ask them who paid them £1700 on that specific date, they will probably tell you, and it will be a fair bet that the name they give you will be will be the beneficial owner of the account, as it is doubtful that he would pay school fees for anybody else". Once again I paused, and then said, "as part of your investigation, shouldn't you have already done all this?" He ignored the question, instead he said

"Tell me again exactly how you came to transfer money, not once, but many times from this account". I patiently went through it again, enumerating each point on my fingers.

"*One…*a prospective client contacts one of our offices, usually Gibraltar, and asks us to incorporate a company for him or her. *Two,* our trained staff ask numerous questions to establish the clients needs."

"What sort of needs would they be?" says macho man…
"Tax evasion"

"Wouldn't that be illegal?" I asked innocently, "No, it could be for many reasons. Asset protection. Collection of royalties. International trading. Legal VAT free trading etc."

"So your office set up the company, then what?"

"Well, let us assume it is the full package. I have already explained exactly what that entails, the office then complete full due diligence enquiries, *including* A DECLARATION OF SOURCE OF FUNDS. When everything is in place the bank account is set up and the client is ready to go. The office provides bank signatories as part of the nominee package. If the client requires a bank transfer carried out, then he must make the request to the office *in writing*. The office will then prepare a transfer request to the bank and pass it on to one of the bank signatories, who may, or may not be me, but would certainly be either a director or a senior manager of the company Being retired, I doubt if I am now signatory for more than half a dozen of the older client accounts, but, having received the form, I would simple sign it and return it to either the office or the bank" Macho man was rapidly writing on a pad. It looked as if it was joined up. "I want to make another point" I said. "I have already told you that the office is licenced under the Financial Services Commission, to obtain a licence is difficult, and one must set many safeguards in place, including a four-eyes policy." He looked up from his joined up writing and said

"four-eyes policy". I nodded; I couldn't believe he needed such basic procedures explained, so I didn't explain them.

"Time for a break" he said suddenly "I'll call the jailer" first of course we had to go through the rigmarole of ending the tapes, taking them out of the machine, labeling them, signing them etc. He then gave me two sheets of paper, neither stabled nor held together with a paper clip, and said.

"I want you to read these carefully, and it may help if you reflect carefully on your position". I took them. The jailer came, took me back to my cell, took my belt, took my shoes, together of course with my dignity, and locked me up. My magazines had gone. But I asked 'My Jailer' if I could have my Caron D'Arche back. He shook his head sadly, and told me it had now been logged in by the custody sergeant, I obviously looked suitably crestfallen, because he rummaged in his pocket and came up with a stub of a pencil with a chewed end. I did not enquire who had done the chewing, but took the stub gratefully, He smiled, perhaps he thought I wanted to write my last will and testament before sticking my head down the concrete toilet and pulling the chain. But nothing was further from my mind; I now had two sheets of paper to read, and two blank sides on which to write. I sat down and started to read the sheets, intending to write up some accurate notes of what had occurred since 8.21 that morning.

The papers dealt with a group of companies, it was obviously the schematic of a carousel, and one of the companies was *Basis Management Limited*. According to the schematic on the paper, *Basis Management* had received, as my son-in-law would have said, '*shed loads of cash*'. It didn't identify individual payments, but the total was quite staggering. Now, the reality was that the schematic showed that Basis Management had received this money, and, I would guess that the bank statements confirmed the amounts. What did appear to be in doubt was whether the source of that money had anything at all to do with a VAT swindle, particularly having identified by one cursory glance at just one of a whole sheath of bank statements, that the thick end of a million pounds had come from a top drawer firm of commercial lawyers. I read each page carefully. There was clearly a link between two of the named company's and Basis Management if the suggestion that money had passed from both the former to the latter was to be believed. I would have to scrutinize the bank statements and have the office identify each payment if I was to be of any help to Macho Man. Now, it has to be said that I had absolutely no desire to help Macho Man, BUT, I did have every intention of helping myself out of my present accommodation, and if that also assisted in the apprehension of a criminal, so much the better. There was a big BUT however. On current showing it did not look as if Macho Man, and presumably his team, would be capable of recognizing a criminal from a loaf of bread. I for sure, and my office without a doubt, would need to be presented with pretty conclusive evidence before they betrayed the confidentiality of a client.

After about one and a half hours the jailer came back for me. It was 5 o'clock, and I had been in custody for eight and a half hours, and now had filled both of my sheets of paper with joined up writing so that Macho Man wouldn't be able to read them IF he made me hand them back to him I was taken back to the interview room for the fourth time in a working day with the thought 'Dosen't time fly when you're having fun'.

"Did you read what I gave you?" said Mach Man - straight in, no messing

"Yes"

"And whom does the account belong to"

"Who, does the account belong to….I have no idea.. BUT, my office will have a complete file with all due diligence"

"You do realize that you are in serious trouble"

"No, what I do realize is that I am in no trouble at all

if you are looking for the *truth*, but a stupidly time wasting short term future if you are simply after a **result**, at any price, and don't intend to let truth, honesty or justice get in the way"

"We know the truth" he said

"Not if it came up and bit you in the soft squidgy bits" I answered. "I can't help recalling this mornings parking ticket" I added. As usual he ignored me, but John graciously cast his eyes to the floor.

"You are familiar with these companies" he said jabbing a copy of the paper I had been given" I said nothing. "I asked you a question" he growled.

"No you didn't" I said, questions usually start with an interrogative. When you start with a command, as you just did it is not a question but a statement, and statements do not require an answer"

"Are you familiar with these companies?" he corrected himself without comment.

"No" only Basis Management"

"Ah so you admit that you know that name"

"Yes, I admit it"

"So how do you know the name?"

"You told it to me about eight hours ago, and have repeated it about one hundred times since. Before this morning I was not familiar with it"

"Tell me about these payments" he handed me a bank statement with a series of payments highlighted in yellow. I looked at them, at first glance there appeared to be a dozen. About five were credits, and seven debits. They came from the two connected companies on the paper I had read, but appeared to have been transferred from various branches of a High Street bank. The seven debits were also to High Street banks, some in the UK, some in other jurisdictions. "Tell me where the money came from, he said, and what checks your company carried out to make sure they were Kosher.

"As you are aware" I said, "I have had no input into the daily affairs of the company since last century". That made him sit up straight, as I thought it would, but I could almost hear the cogs clicking as he slowly worked out that 'last century' was less than seven years ago. I continued "I have no idea what checks my company carried out, but I can state for you the obvious, and tell you what our procedures would have been"

"Now we are getting somewhere"

"We are", I said, "but sadly, as it is the truth so it probably wont be of much help to you." Once again he ignored me...must be page 501 of the little black book on how to ignore a smart-arse. I ran my finger down the figures. "Now then" I said, "in every case the payments appear to have been by electronic transfer. They also appear to have been initiated from major High Street banks" He nodded as if he understood. "They have all been received by Basis Management's bank on the Isle of Man, which is a highly respected private bank, which...I threw this in for good measure....is reputed to be the bankers for the Queen." He didn't nod this time, he probably wasn't quiet sure whether I meant Elizabeth II or Freddie Mercury. The transfers **out** that have been highlighted, may, or may not correspond to the payments **in**. The totals don't appear to tally, but, notwithstanding, they, although not all transferred to UK branches, do all appear to be electronic transfers, once again to well known High Street Banks." There was a bottle of water and a plastic cup on the table, I poured a little and took a sip before continuing. "OK, our checking procedure in this case would have been minimal"

"Are you saying that you wouldn't care where this money came from?"

"Not at all, I am saying that the source of this money would have been checked and re-checked already, several times by people with far greater resources than a small CSP"

"What do you mean?" What do I mean, was this man thick, or was he thick.

"Think about it" I said. "Say Barclays receives in a sum of money from a source, known, or unknown to them, on behalf of a customer, known or unknown to them. Under the KYC *(Know Your Customer)* guidelines of due diligence, they have a responsibility to identify the source of those funds. To make it simple, if I walked into Mr. Barclays with a suitcase containing one million pounds in cash, I would probably be locked in a windowless room while the bank called you guys. If on the other hand Mr. Nat West, sent Mr. Barclay an electronic transfer for one million pounds, Mr. Barclay, may, or may not have instigated his own checks, but most probably he would be quite content in the knowledge that if Mr. NatWest was happy about it, he could be too." I paused to let them catch up. "In other words, I think we can assume that they would both have done their job correctly." Another pause, Macho Man was scribbling furiously. "When", I continued, 'The Queens' bank received the money, they would either have said. '*oh it's come from Barclays, or Nat West, or HSBC so it must be OK*' or they too would have carried out checks, as would the branch of the bank to whom we…"

"To who"

"to **whom**… Bassis Management transferred it. OK, against that background it is highly unlikely that my office would have considered that any source checks would have been necessary, beyond, possibly, having our client sign a standard *declaration of source of funds.*"

"We need to take a break" said Macho Man; "I'll call

the jailer". Once again we went through the rigermarol with the tapes.

Once again we went through the further rigmarole of Belt off, Shoes Off, Dignity…well, as I have already said, that was long gone. I continued writing a chronological account of my day, now *between* the lines of the written side of my two precious pieces of paper. I have to say everybody seemed a little less hostile to me now, and I think that probably, the fact that I had not asked for a lawyer to be present had helped. The fact that I had probably pissed off Macho Man big time, didn't, but you must never forget the old adage.

Big fleas have little fleas

Upon their back to bite 'em,

And so it goes, on and on ……And on

AD INFINITUM

Now I appreciate that the quotation is perhaps not quite right, but, the fact is that there was a time looming large when Macho Man would have to listen to those tapes in the company of his superior officer, and what can one say, when a man keeps his brain in his flack jacket he is in dead trouble when he takes it off. I recorded faithfully all that had happened and waited to be taken back to the interview room. I spent another hour and a half in my little cell, but when I went back the interview had taken on a different tone.

"We want you to write out the alphabet" said Macho Man, giving me a blank sheet of paper and a plastic ball point with yet another chewed end. I contemplated asking if Police Forensics could see if the teeth marks on ball point matched those on the pencil stub. I decided against. I took the paper and handed him back the ball point, carefully avoiding the teeth marks. "I am sure you won't mind me using my own writing instrument" I said, "quietly taking my pencil stub from my top pocket. I think the point was made, and yet another 'smart-arse' point was awarded against me. I wrote out the alphabet in capital letters, saying each letter out loud as I wrote, just in case he didn't recognize them. When I had finished he said

"Now do it again, this time in small letters". I did it again. When I had finished he took the paper and scrutinized it. I am sure that had he been able to count to 26, or indeed known there were 26 letters in the alphabet, he would have checked that they were all there. In the event he actually gave me back the paper, which I must admit included, in both cases, the letter ñ pronounced eña in Spanish, either assuming it was part of the English alphabet, or choosing to ignore it. He then said

"I am now going to read a passage from a book and I want you to write to my dictation." He read an obscure passage about the USSR at the height of its communist strength, about gulags, and community living. I wrote it down faithfully, and gave him back the paper, but not my pencil stub. What did he do, he called the jailer and had me locked up again, although in fairness he did say. "I have to call the jailer again, but I think this is the last time you are going to have to go back to a cell." He could not resist adding….."today." He went on "I have to make a phone call, but I would guess that you will be bailed to present yourself for further questioning in about 9 or 10 weeks." I nodded. I went. He stayed. No more than half an hour passed before the Jailer was back at my front door. He led me back to the interview room that felt like my second home. Macho Man gave me the piece of paper on which I had written out the alphabet….twice. And an obscure and brief treatise of Russian history. He put two new tapes in the machine.

"Did you write this?" he asked.

"Yes" I answered. I was getting too tired to bate him

"Then you would be prepared to sign the paper as being written by you, of your own accord."

"Yes". He passed the paper over to me.

"Sign it" he said "here, and here and here". He pointed to a space under the lower case alphabet, the upper case alphabet and the Russian history. I signed. "Now print your name" he said. I printed my name. "would you agree that you wrote those passages thirty five minutes ago?" He said.

"It feels more like thirty five years" I said, "but if you insist I will accept thirty five minutes."

"OK," he said, "I now need you to date it, write" he looked at his watch "18.25 by the side of it, and initial the date and the time" Poor old Macho Man had obviously had his balls chewed off by his boss *(now then… there's some teeth marks worth checking),* and was now desperate to repair the damage.

"Why?" I said.

"Do you have a problem doing that?" he countered

"Do YOU have a problem with me NOT doing it?" I asked.

"Please sign it" he said. I was so astounded that he knew such a word that I signed it.

"Thank you". Good God, Macho man actually said thank you. He passed me a new blank sheet of paper.

"Now I would like you to write it all down again" he said, and date it, including the time, and sign it".

"Is that the way you were supposed to do it last time?" I asked with a smile. He made no comment. John, who had been a silent witness for hours, suddenly had a coughing fit. What the hell, I wrote it out in LITTLE letters, I wrote it out in BIG letters and I repeated my Russian history.

"Thank you" said Macho man. I smiled as I handed him the paper. "I'm afraid you have to go back into your cell once more" he said, and my office will decide what we have to do" I was locked away for another twenty minutes or so before the jailer came to get me. Macho Man was with him. I imagine that I had got him off a nasty hook with my co-operation, because he was actually very pleasant.

"Look Basil" he said, "I am sorry it has been such a rotten day for you, particularly in view of your health". I couldn't believe it…Macho Man being NICE. He went on "I have good news for you but I have to give it to you in the interview so that everything we say has been recorded on tape"

"What you have just said hasn't been recorded" I said

"I'm sorry, did you speak" he answered. I got the picture. Once more the rigmarole of the tapes. And then.

"Basil Jay, the time is 21.22 and our interview is now being terminated. You will now be taken to the duty officer who will bail you to return to this station on October 18th for further questions which will arise following our ongoing investigations, and interrogation of two lap top and one PC computer removed from your home, together with two mobile phones including one palm top note book, and various files and letters which have been listed and for which we will require you to sign an acknowledgement. After you have been bailed, you will be photographed again, you will be finger printed and a DNA sample will be taken. All of these will be held on a police data base, and will NOT be destroyed irrespective of the outcome of our investigations." He looked at me, and for the very first time there was *almost* a friendly smile on his face "Do you understand?"

"I understand, but think it is disgusting that you can abuse your powers in this way. I am not guilty of anything. In the fullness of time that will become evident to you all, and, of course, I will be un-arrested – or whatever you call it technically. BUT you are saying that my fingerprints, photograph and DNA will, notwithstanding, will be held on police data bases for ever more"

"That is the position" he said. I was bailed, I was fingerprinted, I was photographed, and I had a DNA swab taken. They then took me home. As we arrived in my drive way, I said, and hoped they would not miss the sarcasm.

"I want to thank you both for the deep courtesy that you have shown me today" They were silent. I think they missed the sarcasm. Macho Man turned to me and had the cheek to say,

"To be honest Basil, we didn't think you were going to be involved right from the beginning" Oh I said, believing that he would then confide that I had an honest face…not a bit of it, instead he said.

"When we picked up Mark Southerby, we drove down a long drive to a huge and impressive country house. In the drive was an Aston Martin, and in the garage, which had been converted from a one time barn, was a Bentley and a Range Rover". He had a safe as well….but the money in inside was *not* Zimbabwean. He paused and actually smiled again "Mark Southerby gave the impression of having had his fingers in a £50m pie" He pointed at my own stately pile, with Polly's three or four year old Peugeot 206 Cabriolet standing in the drive. "Nice little house", he said, "handy little run-a-bout" he had the affrontery to pat me on the shoulder. "Nuff said" He grinned. Macho Man had got in the last word

As I rang my doorbell *(I had no keys of course)* Polly opened the door. I had been in custody for more than thirteen hours. Polly had been home for two or three hours and had spent over ten hours in custody. She had gone through exactly the same procedures. There was one interesting point. When she arrived home the search team were waiting for her *(she had no keys either)* .They had searched thoroughly and carried away a huge amount of personal items. BUT, it had obviously become clear to the search team quite early on, that this was a mistake. They found nothing incriminating because there was nothing incriminating to find. They had conducted a thorough search with great restraint. Everything was as tidy as it had been before they arrived. The leader of the search team actually had the decency to say to Polly. "Mrs. Jay, I am sorry about the upheaval, we have been very careful and have tidied up after us." She thanked them. They gave her a huge list of the items taken. And they were gone. What were my first words when I got in the house? Predictably.

"Get your coat on Polly, let us go and have a good meal, a good bottle of wine, a G & T or two, and reflect on yet another golden thread that has been woven into the rich tapestry that has been our lives." I went to get my wallet from the drawer of the bedside cabinet. It was missing, as indeed were both of our passports. *Luckily* we did still have almost three million Zimbabwean dollars in the safe without a key, but more importantly we had a rapport with our local restaurant which meant that we could always, go late, forget our wallet and purse, have a good meal, and pay the tab later. However, ALL of this had happened on a Thursday morning. Luckily Polly had had the sense to insist on a lawyer. The next morning, Friday, the lawyer called Macho Man, who, would you believe, had actually given me his business card when we had parted company the previous night. He hadn't said, but clearly implied *"Here you are Basil, if you ever have a friend who would like to be shouted at 300 decibels, just have him give me a call"*) However, his card enabled Polly's lawyer to telephone, explain to him that he had no rights to take my wallet, my credit cars, my driving licence, my passport, and my membership card to the 'Blue Angel' club in Frith Street, Soho, and that HE, the lawyer wanted them back pronto, because his client was going to Tenerife on the following day *(which was true)* and his client's husband owed a restaurant bill from the night before *(which was also true)*. In any event, Macho man told him he could POP UP TO LONDON *(a round trip of about two and a half hours)* and collect them. He did so; I collected them all from his home that Friday evening, and reflected on the stupidly draconian powers of a half-a-brain megalomaniac.

The next morning, our very good friends and neighbours knocked on our door. "How are you both?" said Pauline, "we have been so worried, we saw you *'leaving the house with your friends yesterday'*, and then there were men everywhere. What an earth has happened?" Polly, thinking on her feet, gave Harry and Pauline a big smile and said.

"Oh, no, everything is fine WE'VE HAD THE BUILDERS IN"

Polly is one of the most honest people I know *(I, of course, come a very close second)*, but even with this knowledge our lovely neighbours had obviously found it very hard to accept that we had managed to find a co-operating team of builders called '**POLICE',** and '**CUSTOMS AND EXCISE',** who, in addition to their strange names, had opted to replace the traditional 'hard hats' of the jobbing builder with the, less traditional, blue flack jackets and holstered revolvers.

After a day or so we were invited to join our friends 'for a drink, and a few nibbles'. Harry and Pauline had also had the foresight to invite two other close neighbours and friends. Once we were settled with our Gin and Tonics in their comfortable conservatory overlooking their delightful English country garden with the, still warming, rays of the late July sun beaming through the windows, Pauline, by way of small talk, delicately touched upon the question uppermost in their collective minds.

"OK, you two. Tell us all about your *builders*". We told them about the builders. I told my story, which you have now all heard, and then Polly told hers.

A NOTE FOR THE RECORD. On September the 20^{th,} Polly received a letter telling her that she would not be required to answer Bail. I had to wait a lot longer, because I had not received such a letter by October 8th; I was already in Tenerife by that time. Nevertheless, I had telephoned the police station to confirm the time that I had to present myself on the 18th, and had been told that there appeared to be no requirement for me to present myself on that, or as far as they knew, any other day, but I would, no doubt, be told if the position changed. It was not, however until April 30th (NINE MONTHS) after the events outlined above, that I received a letter saying that having completed their investigation, NO PROSECUTION WAS CONSIDERED NECCESSARY. And later a further letter asking me to **make the appropriate arrangements to GO TO LONDON TO COLLECT THE ITEMS THAT WERE SEIZED IN THE SEARCH.** *No apology. No explanation. No information. In the end, Macho Man* **HAD** *won.*

CHAPTER 9

A MATTER OF PERSPECTIVE

Now I am not going to suggest that I had been shackled to a wall during that July experience, I had no electrodes attached to my dangly-down bits. Were the soles of my feet beaten with a rubber hose pipe? No, they were not. Macho Man might have been loud, he might have been un-pleasant, he might have been a grade-one pratt, but my thirteen plus hours under his tender administrations were hardly life-threatening. And yet, you know, for many months afterwards it rankled that the thick end *(not the thickest end, because he was in the cell with me at the police station)* of a dozen police and customs officers spent the whole day in my home. Going through cupboards, opening drawers, looking through private files, reading personal letters, and in the end taking away two mobile phones, two computers, bank and credit card statements, company board minutes and investment plans. I still wake in the middle of the some nights and almost scream at the injustice of it, of the unnecessary intrusion into my privacy. But then an event happened that made me realize it was all meaningless....*it was all a matter of perspective.*

Through the first of my 'Tigers' books Polly and I had met up again with very close friends from our children's *'growing-up'* years. Friends of over 40 years who we have not seen since I retired to the Isle of Man in 1990. We invited them to visit us in our Tenerife home, and, in October 2006, we had a wonderfully nostalgic week. Over dinner one evening I had regaled them with the story of our arrest, much as you have read it. They were devastated that we had been through so much, and eventually the talk turned away from the unpleasantness of life and to the times when we were all young, and beautiful and living in Bexhill-On-Sea. Because, indeed Marjorie had brought with her proof that such was once the case, providing always that one never loses sight of the old adage, *'beauty is in the eye of the beholder'* and when looking at *my* photograph I *was* the beholder, and *I* thought I looked both young and….well you know where I'm at.. I had in my hand a photograph of a dinner party at our wonderful old house The Thorne. WOW, were we really so young, and, as a group, so attractive. Could that really be me, slim and fit, masses of dark brown hair, and a smile I used my own teeth for. It must have been about 1977. There was a lump in my throat as I looked at those dear friends. We would be in our mid- thirties. There was Roger, an accountant and Assistant County Treasurer, we played squash together and we played cricket together.

"It is just wonderful to have you both here" I said to John and Marjorie, "I tapped the photo, what's old Roger doing with himself these days. I expect he retired at about 55 with small pot of gold from the tax payer". Marjorie was quiet for a moment.

"Roger died two years ago of a thrombosis" she said, "He had had a leg amputated and was recovering well, but then he relapsed and died". I almost could not believe what I was hearing. I tapped another face in the photograph.

"How is David" I asked, looking at the smiling face of our friend, and for me business associate. An Architect with whom I had prepared many projects.

"David's fine", said John, although we don't see an awful lot of him these days, he's married again and lives out in the country. That was better.

"What about Terry" I said, flicking the picture with my finger, is he still in the village taking things easy.

"Terry died last year of lung cancer" said John. "We were at his birthday party just before Christmas and he was not feeling too well, he went to the doctors and they diagnosed lung cancer. It was inoperable, and he died within two months" - speechless. "He never ever smoked, you know" John finished quietly.

I looked again at the photograph in my hand, I would guess that I was about 35; Polly of course is a little younger. It must have been just a year or two after we returned from our Indian trip. There was Malcolm, our doctor and a very dear friend, and his wife Jan, one of the loveliest ladies I have ever known, even though she was a JP. Our daughter, who would have been around seven at the time, once caused great hilarity amongst our friends, and gossip amongst those who knew us by name only. Polly had been into hospital to have a very nasty operation, a laminectomy, where a disc is removed from the spine. She was in hospital a week or two, and told to take it easy when she went home. Our friendly doctor, Malcolm knew that my expertise lay outside of the house with such implements as Hoovers, Dusters, and Brooms being quite alien to me. He very kindly therefore invited us both to spend a week with him and Jan as a start to the convalescence. Our children were staying with my mother, and she was happy to keep them for an extra week. At school one morning, Tania's teacher asked "And how is your mother dear" to which Tania replied.

"Mummy's gone to live with Dr. Wicks. I received many a strange glance until the truth became known. But, back to our photo album. There is John R, our solicitor and friend, who always steered me out of trouble (of the commercial kind), or if I had put myself in it, got me out again. There was his wife Paddy. A treasure, a choreographer, and a wonderful friend. There was David F, my architect of a hundred projects and his wife Chris. We became very quiet as it hit home that around that happy dinner table of thirty-somethings, no less than five of them were no longer with us. Roger …. dead. Terry ….. Dead.

David B, husband of Janice who taught our daughter to dance…dead. Patrick, with who I shared so many 'young developers' dreams……… dead. Albert, a little older than us, but a font of practical wisdom. Dead. Dear Lord, what a hand we have drawn, and how lucky we are still to be breathing God's air, and playing Golf Del Sur's golf course.

We opened a new bottle of Moet et Chandon, and toasted absent friends with a lump in our throats.

Macho Man became just an insignificant bit part of my life, a single day, a single day of a life that had enjoyed so much and had to endure so little.

CHAPTER 10

CHAPTER ONE RE-VISITED

Basil, I have great news for you" I looked into the beaming face of the lovely Nita. "I now have the result of your body scan, your bone scan, your cat scan, your lab test, your liver scan, your abdominal scan, your ECG, all 233 of your blood tests, your glucose tolerance test, your doctor tolerance test, your liver function test, your kidney function test, your eye test, and even your driving test, and I can tell you with absolute certainty that THEY HAVE FOUND ABSOLUTELY NOTHING WRONG - *with the little toe on your left foot,*" She smiled winningly, "the rest of you is falling apart, but that little toe" she paused...."wow". My gaze dropped to the beautiful pink fluffy 'elephant ears' slippers she was wearing, and then back to her face which had now changed into Homer Simpson's wife with her blue hair piled so high that it was almost touching the ceiling.

"Basil, you have gone very quiet, you seem to be in a world of your own" I spun around at the sound of the voice, there peering around the green folding screen in the corner of the room (where she had gone to some time earlier to '*phone the family'*) was the lovely Nita, In a world of my own, I had of course been, a place I had been increasingly visiting of recent months. I looked at her "Sorry Nita, I said", and to lighten the tone "I must have dozed off"

"That's OK, she answered, I'm nearly ready to take a couple of gallons of blood for analysis". I have to say, that the last ten or fifteen minutes or so had been such a harrowing journey through my memory that I had almost lost the plot.

My first feeling was one of relief that she no longer looked like Homer Simpson *(or his wife)* and had regained her usual physiognomy, whilst her pink elephant ear slippers had converted into a pair of sensible shoes.

"Who are *you?*" I asked.

"I am the silly GP who should know better to waste her time, even on an enigma, such as you" but she was smiling, and because she was smiling, I thanked her profusely,

"There is no need to thank my profusely" I imagined her saying, "it is all part of the service" She folded back the wheeled screen and came and stood next to me. "I just need about 10 minutes to shut up shop" she quietly burst into that old Frank Sinatra classic "There's no-one in the place except you and me" No she didn't, but by her smile she certainly implied exactly that sentiment.

"Now then she said, you just relax and reflect on the winter behind you, and then I will be back before you know it to take the first steps to putting your mind at rest" I smiled a thank you, she smiled a 'sit tight for a moment' smile back and went out of the door, through which, a hundred years earlier a clot had entered.

I closed my eyes, and, as I had been told, I reflected on the winter now gone.

Our winter had passed by at its usual slow and delightful

pace. Polly and I usually rose at the crack of 10 o'clock at times having had, what I called, '*essential practice to overcome my current difficulties*', and what she called a '*romantic interlude .... but quick before the toast burns*' We generally had our breakfast on the sun-drenched terraced overlooking the sixth fairway of our Tenerife golf club. On Monday we would wander down to the first tee for mid-day to take part in the weekly scramble. On Tuesday, it would be a day of rest. Following our leisurely breakfast we would aim the car up into the mountains for one of our favoured lunchtime bistros. Restaurante El Mirador in Villaflora *(The highest village in Spain)* or Cerres de Luna in Camella. On Wednesday, after we had broken our fast, we would toddle down to the first tee for the weekly Taboos mixed FBBB. And then on Thursday it was MY day of rest whilst Polly played in ladies day. Special responsibilities this year of course, being Lady Captain. Friday was my favourite golf day of the week with our regular Swallow's competition, followed always by a typically Canarian meal in a typical Canarian restaurant. As many as 60 of us for much of the winter season. And then the restful week-end, where usually we would just do nothing......and if we hadn't finished doing that by lunchtime, we would carry on during the afternoon, after we had had a long lunch in the sunshine.

It must be said, that in the 16 weeks before Christmas we had visiting friends for about nine of them, but every 'Swallow's' friend soon becomes a friend of every 'Swallow' and our days, our lunches, or evening meals al fresco, our parties and our musical soirees become a life just so different from that which a Swallow spends when he returns to the UK for the summer. Already my hospital summer was a faded memory, and sometimes I would go as much as five minutes without even thinking about Macho-Man

During my lazy winter, Sharron my business partner

had been very very busy in Bulgaria. She had kept me in the loop by email and I had got to know the sorts of deals she was looking at and the sorts of properties she was buying and refurbishing. She had created a wonderful rapport with the Mayor of one of the larger Municipalities in the Southern Region of Bulgaria. It had been about October time when she had telephoned me and said. "Hello Boss", she always called me that although it had long since ceased to be true "What do you know about building a golf course?". Of course, I had no option to be anything but scrupulously honest.

"There's not much anyone can teach me", I said, "about building a Golf Course."

"Great" she said, "How many square metres do we need?"

"I'll get back to you " I said

"How many properties do we need around the course to make it viable?" she said

"I'll get back to you" I said

"What does it cost to build 18 holes?" she paused, "or would you rather get back to me" she said, A bright girl is Sharron.

Luckily, I didn't get where I am today without knowing people who know more than I do, and a few phone calls later I knew we needed about 150 acres for a golf course, and at least 500 properties to make it a truly profitable venture. This of course meant a further 50 acres or so of land. So I was able to phone Sharron back within a day or two.

"Hi Sharron" I started, I have been giving some thought to your golf course, and I think I have the answers for you."

"You mean you've been phoning around" she said with a chuckle. I took a leaf out of Macho Man's book and ignored her.

"For the golf course you need a minimum of 150 acres, that's……"

"About 600,000 square metres" she finished for me.

About 600,000 square metres I agreed. "Then you need at least a further 50 acres….."

"200,000 square metres" she said

"200,000 square metres" I agreed, "for the housing"

"That's a total of 800,000 square metres I said.

"I've already told Gicho that we would need about one and a half million square metres" she said, "and he's…."

"Who is Gicho?" I asked,

"The Mayor" she said, "and he's….."

"getting back to you" I said, playing her at her own game

"short listed four sites for us to look at" she continued, starting a new game of her own.

"When?" I asked

"Not before the end of January" she said "apparently when the old regime was overthrown, people who had had land seized by the state were given 15 years to claim it back. Any land not so claimed becomes the property of the state on January 31st next year"

She gave me a moment to catch up before continuing "Gicho has obviously earmarked the sites, but does not want to us to view or to commit until after the deadline in case a legitmate owner puts in a claim."

"That's less than three months away" I said

"I had worked that out" Sharron replied.

And so, Christmas came and Christmas went. And then one day, in January, a phone call, "Hello Boss, I've been talking to Gicho"

"And?"

"We can look at three of the four sites he talked about, but one is now a no no"

"When can we see them?"

"Can you get to Bulgaria next week?"

"I can, but Polly can't, lady captains duties and all that"

"Gicho wants us to make a decision, and you know how you said we needed 500 properties to make it pay"

"Yes"

"Well, I told Gicho we wouldn't consider any deal less than TWO golf course and............"

"and what?"

"and 3,000 properties"

"What did he say?"

"He has offered us 2,500,000 square metres on the edge of a beautiful village called Alexandrovo."

"That's nearly 600 acres" I cut in

"I know" she answered

"Anyway, if the site is suitable he will get the wheels moving"

"Wow" I said, 2,500,000 square metres of land on wheels, we can move it where we like."

"Very funny...anyway boss, are you available?"

"Of course I am, ready, willing, and able". Little did I know that that decision would lead to my hurling myself down one of the longest escalators in Gatwick Airport. But I have explained all of that.

After the blood covered, upgraded, hostess pampered, flight from Gatwick to Tenerife I had been met at the airport by Polly, who, luckily, on account of the fact that I was wearing a black shirt, was not immediately aware of the, non to subtle, blood colouring around the collar and shoulders of the shirt, although, she did comment on the fact that I had a plaster on my ear. In any event, our chat between the Rena Sofia airport in Tenerife Sur and our home on Golf Del Sur, was about how Bulgaria was looking, and did we find any sites that appealed to us. The fact was, that the one we had looked at in the small village of Alexandrovo was more than perfect. Alexandrovo literally means 'Place of Alexander'. The story is that when he was busy conquering the then known world, he made a fortress in Alexandrovo whilst he brought the Bulgars and the Tartars to heel. This beautiful small village is approached by a 7km long Roman Road which was as straight as a die, and bordered by wild roses. The village is small, just 300 houses and 400 or 500 souls, all of whom were either over 70 or under 10.

Grandparents looking after children whilst parents travelled many miles and lived away from home in order to find work. The land, like Topsy just grew and grew and the area we were now being offered extended to 4,500,000 square metres. Over 1200 acres, and we knew that if we could secure it and develop it as we wanted, we would bring a new wealth and prosperity to Alexandrovo beyond their wildest dreams *(and it wouldn't do us any harm either)*

But, that was still in the future. AND suddenly I was brought back to the present. The lovely Nita, had , I assumed, listened to my earlier update without dozing off, although I couldn't be certain because I had not been able to see behind the screen where she had gone to '*phone the family*' Anyway, now she was back…syringe in her hand..

"OK Basil, thanks for up-dating me, I have quietened the braying brood at home, and locked up for the night. But I would still like to get home in time for the Epilogue, so lets just take a couple of pints of blood and arrange for a scan or three, and then we can set about sorting you out.

She tapped away on her keyboard "a letter" she said to "your consultant, to arrange some more scans…he will probably want to see you again first" I just smiled; I really did not mind the prospect of seeing Dr D again. "Now" she said "lets have your left arm, that's good, now clench and unclench a fist for me… perfect…. You will just feel a little scratch" I grinned at her, she grinned back, I am sure we were both remembering the pre-PC days, when she would have said "You will just feel a little prick", and I would have made an appropriate reply. Ahh, such were the days, when children could climb trees and throw sticks up at the conkers. "OK, Basil, all done…. The blood test will be back in about 3 days…I will give you a call"

"Thank you Nita" I said… "for everything"

"Let me let you out she said" she did, and I drove meditatively back to Polly.

A good as her word, 3 days after the blood was taken, the surgery telephoned. It was Joan, the secretary. "Hello Mr Jay" she said, "Dr. Hakelin is in surgery but has asked me to call you to arrange a *double* appointment for Friday. Will you be able to pop in at 9.30?" I knew there was no point in quizzing Joan, so I simple said,

"OK Joan, I will be there" ….and I was

On Friday I sat in the waiting room with Polly. The wall computer gave me the news. "BASIL JAY TO ROOM 7" I went to room 7 and knocked.

"Come in"

"I went in"

"Basil"

"And Mrs Basil" I said

"And Mrs Basil…welcome, but to what do I owe the pleasure"

"Well, I was told to make a DOUBLE appointment, and as Polly wasn't doing anything I thought I would bring her along"

"I see Basil….well, I am glad to see you are still taking everything so seriously" I smiled to show her that I wasn't. "You are not the most uncomplex patient I have"

"Uncomplex"

"Uncomplex…it is a word isn't it?" I scratched my head

"Well", I said, in the same way I suppose that you can UNlose your car keys when you find them, or be UN arrested for a crime when you are found to have been in the shower with the all England ladies cricket team at the time of the incident, so yes…we'll go along with UNcomplex"

"Literary bighead" she said, I just grinned, and Polly stayed silent, she had sat through my pedantic tormenting before.

"Sorry, I said, but in what way am I NOT UN" she put her head on one side and looked at me like a person with her head on one side.

"NOT UN" she said,

"You said", I said, "I was Not UNcomplex, I assume that to mean that you think I am complex"

"Well" said the lovely Nita, "most patients come into my surgery, and they have, a cough, or a cold, or a hernia, or stomache ache, which they got by eating something that disagreed with them" she paused, as if preparing for the good bit, "you on the other hand present a fistful of symptoms before me, having acquired them as a result of having thrown yourself down an escalator at Gatwick Airport" she was ready for the 'punch line'

"You, Basil….are NOT UNcomplex". I was disappointed

"Does that mean I'm not an enigma any more?" I asked, the lovely Nita ignored me, she was obviously outside of her comfort zone and anxious to get back to the safety of medical diagnosis.

Well", she said, "YOU have got" she began counting off on her fingers ONE "high blood pressure, TWO high cholesterol, THREE your plasma gamma is high, FOUR your hemoglobin is high, FIVE your AST is high, SIX your blood sugar, well we will come to that in a minute, SEVEN you've got arthritis in the feet, EIGHT you've got arthritis in your thumb, NINE you say you might have a hernia", She leaned back in her chair. "You'll be telling me you've got piles next", she said with grin that could have munched a thousand chips.

"Piles of what?" I asked, po-faced. She swallowed the last of the chips and got serious.

"Basil, the one thing you don't seem to suffer from is 'Stress BUT'" she sat quietly as the corners of her mouth slowly turned up at the same time as my toes. "By golly, you're a carrier" the dénouement was out, the day had been won, the Doctor had reigned supreme and it was now time to get serious…she said

"I have the unhappy result of your glucose tolerance test"

"Is that why we have a DOUBLE appointment?" I asked

"There is a lot to explain" she explained

"You better explain then" I exclaimed

"I don't claim to be an expert on diabetes" she continued, "but we do have a diabetic expert in the practice…her name is Karen" she paused.

"Karen" I said, feeling a need to fill the gap.

"Karen" she repeated, "and today, if you are not busy, I am going to make a Doctor Day." She waited for me to object. I stayed silent. She looked at her computer screen. "You," she said, in an 'it serves you jolly well right sort of a voice' "are paying the price of avoiding the English winter by sunning yourself on a Tenerifian beach"

"Don't do beaches" I said

"Don't be pedantic" she replied, before continuing, "most patients can spread their appointments over a longer period, whereas we have to squeeze yours into a" she searched for a suitable expression, "a small window of opportunity" I helped her out

"a limited window of opportunity" she re-fined, "so **this** is what you are going to do" she waited for me to respond, but I kept mum – although of course, mum would have denied it. "it is now 10.05 and you have been sitting at my desk for almost 10 minutes." She tapped on her computer keyboard. Sister has a slot at 10.30 at Harrietsham" lucky sister, I thought, but said nothing. "I have just booked you in for a multiple blood test which goes beyond the one I have the results of here, and enables us to measure your average blood performance over the past three months." I waited for Polly to say

"Have you got a test for bedroom performance" but she remained silent......clearly well satisfied, or am I having a touch of male ego massage. The lovely Nita was speaking again.

"Obviously we cannot use such a test for diagnostic purposes, but it is quite acceptable as a monitoring tool". She hardly paused for breath. "Then, at 4.30 you are going to see Karen who is the practice diabetic specialist. With Karen I have booked you a DOUBLE appointment"

"a DOUBLE" I began, "so I better take...."

"Your wife" she finished for me", then added, that was actually quite funny" she paused....."the FIRST time" she finished. "Do you realize that, since you got back from Tenerife, just two weeks ago, you have had NINE, yes NINE appointments either here with me, with the practice nurses, or with the Hospital?"

"Wow" I said

"And it is far from over yet," she said. "Over the next two weeks you are going to see the Dr Lypin who is a specialist in Metabolic Medicine and a Consultant in Chemical Pathology. She is going to assess you, and hopefully produce a definitive balance diet of drugs and medicines."

"Dr Lypin" I said

"You are going to see Toni Wagner, who is a Cardio Specialist nurse in the Cardio Respiratory Department, where, you will have a series of ECG's between which you will walk, run, hop, and probably collapse on a treadmill.

"Like the little white mice" I asked. Nita chose not to answer.

"You are then coming back to see me, when I want to decide whether to start you off on an ACE inhibitor, AND start regular renal monitoring. You then have an appointment with Dr Alonso about your predication to sunburned lip0s which won't heal, and finally you are back with Dr Henry Draper to investigate why your PSA has started rising again FOR THE THIRD TIME". Like an underwater archeologist she had to pause for breath. She continued. "By my calculations that will be a total of THIRTEEN medical appointments in 28 days, which, if you take out Christmas, the New year, and Week-ends is THIRTEEN appointments NINETEEN working days"

"Am I still an enigma?" I asked

"Oh no, I think I have solved the mystery that was Basil" she smiled, "I think you are just gathering material for you next book"

"What, this one?" I asked

"Which one" she said. I smiled, because I knew something that she didn't....and I was not alone.....was I? However, before I left I needed a little a bit of medical information, to say nothing of the last word.

"Nita" I said, I have had diagnosed Arf-ritis for about ten years. I have had operations on my foot and my hand to remove, or fuse bones. My question is this, how long do I have to wait before my **ARF-** ritis becomes **FULL-** ritis? "

"Get out of my surgery" she, said and go and annoy Sister at Harrietsham"

CHAPTER 11

THE SCARY LADY

Before Christmas I had managed to see Sister in Harrietsham, I had seen Karen the Diabetic Specialist, and I had listened carefully to the instructions imparted by both… However there was one appointment which had to be delayed until after the festive season. In the event I was grateful that I had had the chance to stoke up the inner fires before coming face to face with the doctor who will always been known in the Jay household, as 'Scary Lady', a doctor in whose company I became quipless. Dr. YY Lypin was totally without Ruth, but as time went on I was to appreciate beyond measure that measureless ruthlessness.

Dr Y.Y. Lypin turned out to be a lady of, what one always politely refers to as 'uncertain age'. I however, had no problem in narrowing the range. I was certain that she was somewhere between 40 and 60. Tall, a big woman – not overweight, just, statuesque, even majestically matronly.

She had walked into the waiting room of the Newfields Private Hospital in Royal Tunbridge Wells, a waiting room into which I had arrived early for my appointment, and was half way through my second cup of cappuccino. Having, I must say, carelessly, albeit unintentionally, thrown three-quarters of the first cup over a 'decade old' issue of Kent Life, the plastic chair I was about to sit on, and the floor in that order. It was only remarkable dexterity on my part that allowed me to rescue the remaining contents of the cup before filling it, once more to the brim, I had started to ineffectually dab at the dampness on seat and floor, when a fortuitously passing hospital orderly with a mop and bucket said.

"That's OK, leave it to me". I left it to him.

"Basil Jay" boomed a vaguely Teutonic voice. I looked up towards the reception desk where this tall lady in twin set and pearls was glancing around the room as if trying to decide who could possibly be the individual brave enough to impose upon her time on a Monday morning in mid January. I placed my cup and saucer on top of a still damp copy of Kent Life, and stood.

"That's me" I said in a thin voice, and then strengthened it with an "over here". She loosely extended her arm and beckoned me towards her as she turned away and began to stride purposefully toward her room.

"Follow me" spoken over her shoulder. What else could I do, I followed her. We passed through a set of double doors and then into a room with the name Dr YY Lypin on the door. She did not hold it open for me, but relied on, what she had obviously instantly recognized as my lightning fast reflexes, probably as a result of the dexterity she had witnessed in the episode of the cup of cappuccino. In that act she had surely decided that I had ample ability to catch the door before it flattened my nose.

"Shut the door and sit down" she said. I shut the door and stood where I was. A small act of defiance but one that I thought was important just to show who was paying who.

"Sit down" she said sharply. I sat down.

She crossed one long, once shapely leg (and I have to say still pretty shapely), over the other, her sensible skirt, insensibly rode up to mid thigh giving me a fairly extensive view of white, probably once irresistible flesh, *(and I have to say, still not bad when viewed by a man of 'uncertain age')* before flicking her long blonde hair over her shoulder with splayed fingers. Her chair was next to mine. I sat in front of her desk, but she sat, not behind it, but almost beside me at its corner. She leaned forward slightly and said.

"First, answer these questions" The phrase, *'Ve 'ave' ze vays of making you talk'* ran through my mind but I pushed it to one side and concentrated on the still partly revealed lower thigh.

"You are Basil Jay" my normally flippant response of 'I know' did not seem appropriate, or even safe.

"Yes" I said instead.

"You are 65 years old"

"Yes"

"You were born on 28th July 1942"

"Yes", at another time I would have suggested these were statements rather than questions; BUT as Dr YY Lypin was far scarier than Macho Man, I kept silent.

"You had a radical prostatectomy in 2004"

"Yes"

"When you were 62"

"That's right" no-one was going to call me a 'yes man'

"In February 2006 your PSA began to rise"

"Yes, from 0.1, to 0.4 and then to 0.7"

"So you were put on to a course of Hormone Therapy"

"I was"

"Is that when you began to put on weight?"

"Yes"

"That was followed by Radiation Therapy"

"Correct"

"Any side effects?"

"Apart from the weight gain, no"

"Why do you think your GP has sent you to see me?" ah!, I thought, a real life question at last. "I'll tell you" she said before I could answer. Not a question after all, I thought, she continued "she sent you to see me because you would appear to be in danger of liver damage.

"Oh…..is it really bad?" I ventured.

"Not yet, but, in the last few months your LFTs have become abnormal, and a recent liver ultrasound showed a fatty liver"

"Oh" I said

"I have reviewed all of your results on the computer" she continued, "let me tell *you* what it tells *me* about *you*" I so wanted to say to her,

"I just love it when you talk pro-nouns", But, unlike the lovely Nita, I did not think she was ready for role play. Instead she proceeded to tell me what it told her about me, and, if I had understood it I am sure it would not have made pretty listening…..and although listen I did, understand I did not. You will therefore be forgiven if you skip the next couple of paragraphs. 'Scary Lady' had already launched into seemingly scary statistics.

"In 2004" she said, "your cholesterol was 8.2 mmo/l triglycerides 1.9mmol/L, HDL 1.5mmol/L 5.8 mmol/L". She looked me straight in the eyes as if inviting me to contradict her.

"Wow" was all I could think to say.

"In September 2004 your lipids had improved, AST was slightly raised at 39/UL" she paused. I looked blank "The reference range is 10/34 U/L" she said.

"Ouch" I replied.

"IN March 2005 LFTs were normal, as they were still

in September. Your lipids were then quite satisfactory with a cholesterol of 4.6 mmol/L, triglycerides 1.3 mmol/L, HDL 1.5 mmol/L, and LDL 2.5 mmol/L

"That's comforting" I felt the need to offer.

"BUT" isn't there just *always a BUT*. "By December 2006 your AST had increased to 48 U/L. *AND* your lipids had deteriorated"

"Damned lipids" I said, with a grin. The grin fell on stony features. She carried on like a bulldozer at a demolition derby.

"Things were going from bad to worse. By September 2007 AST was 107 U/L and by November 2007 it was 255 U/L" she paused, and then reminded me of the normal range. She paused to take a breath, and then, "let me remind you" she said, "that the normal range for AST is 10 to 34. Also, your gamma GT was 312 IU/L. HOWEVER" I feared the worse, but things appeared to be slightly improving "in December 2007 your AST had decreased to 115 U/L"

"Oh goody" I thought, but my joy was to be short lived.

""But on the 3rd January 2008 it had slightly increased to 123 U/L AND FURTHERMORE", If it isn't a BUT, it's a bloody FURTHERMORE. "your Gamma GT had increased to 355 IU/L"

She sat back in her chair for all the world as if she had just completed the balcony scene from Romeo and Juliet. She waited for me to speak.

"Thank you for that run down" I said, feeling as if I had been 'run down' "I didn't understand a lot of it but the main thrust would suggest that something is not going according to plan, at least", I managed one of my cynical smiles, "certainly not any *earthly* plan"

"Do you smoke?" she said, taking me by surprise

"I gave up on August 1st 1971 at approximately 9pm

in the evening" I said, proving that I to had total recall of things that were, what I call, 'notables' in my life.

"How can you be so precise?" she asked.

"Well", I began, "a GP, in fact a locum standing in for a good GP friend of mine, was called to my bedside because I had bronchitis and was having difficulty getting my breath. He was shown up to the bedroom, but didn't come in, but leaning on the door jamb he simply said.

"I heard you wheezing as I was coming up the stairs" I wheezed a gentle 'oh! at him. "You obviously smoke" he said from his place on the door jamb, "how many cigarettes a day do you smoke?"

"I do", I said thinking at the same time that that would be a good line for a wedding, then collecting my thoughts continued.

"Between 40 *wheeze* and 60 *wheeze* a day"

"Between" he glared, "What does that range depend on?"

"It depends" I wheezed, "on whether I smoke *wheeze* 40 or *wheeze* 60 on any given day". I waited for him to chortle at my clever retort in the face of wheezing adversity. He just ran his fingers through his bushy beard, but remained totally without chortle.

"I can do nothing for you", he said, pushing himself off the door jamb.

"I could almost hear your chest from the front door." He appeared to change the subject.

"How long have you been unable to work?" he said.

"About six weeks", said Polly, clearly on my side.

"Listen" he said, "This bout of bronchitis will probably see you off work for about three months, within five or six years you probably will not be able to work at all.

"My advice" he had said, "is never to smoke again" I never smoked again. I was 29 years old

"Good" said the good Dr. YY Lypin."That shows you have will power" she paused before adding "and you are going to need it"

"Of course, I'm sure it will be in a good cause" I said.

"Depends", she said with a steely glare, "whether or not you think staying alive is a good cause" she very lightly prodded my shoulder with her finger. Then she changed her theme.

"I am told you live in Tenerife during the winter"

"I do", I said, hoping to warm to the subject.

"I expect as an ex-pat you drink too much", I was about to give my stock answer of 'I'm only a social drinker' when she said "and don't give me any of that guff about just being a social drinker, just tell me how many units you drink each week."

"About 50….or so" I said" Somehow I couldn't dredge up the courage to be economical with the truth.

"Harrumph", she said "I suggest that you are being somewhat economical with the truth" I sort of shrugged. "You know you have now been diagnosed with diabetes" she said, moving swiftly on, "do you know what that means?"

"vaguely" I said

"Well I'll tell you *'precisely'*" she replied.

"Pretty much everything you eat is being turned to sugar, and your body, is unable to process that sugar in the normal way. The result is it turns to fat". Before I could respond she asked me "How much weight have you put on since you had your radical prostatectomy?"

"About two and a half stone" I said.

"Not surprised," she went on, "some of it was as a result of the hormone therapy. Particularly the breasts" She looked at mine pointedly, I did my best **not** to repay the compliment – but failed. "The rest is the sugar to fat problem. I am now going to give you a thorough examination and then tell why you are going to need all the will power you have for the next four weeks."

I stripped of my shirt and lay on the couch. She prodded my stomach and said "that is what we call 'bad fat'. What we call 'Prominent Central Obesity – or PCO" she continued to knead and prod "You have a soft and enlarged liver, but the scan had revealed no other liver stigmata - yet, nor lipid stigmata. You are, what we call, clinically euthyroid. I am going to take your blood pressure", she took my blood pressure. "Not good," she said "170/110, AND you have an irregular pulse. BUT, your chest is clear and your heart sounds normal. You can put your shirt on now." I heaved my prominent central obesity – or PCO, off the couch and put my shirt back on. As I was doing so she said,

"a number of things can affect your liver to a stage where it first becomes 'fatty' but ultimately can lead to serious liver disease. By now I had tucked my shirt in and sat down in front of her again. "Prominent Central Obesity"

"PCO" I helped out

"PCO", she agreed gentle prodding my own personal PCO with her index finger "is the worst thing for your liver, but some statins and alcohol also can do considerable damage". I could think of nothing to say so I said nothing, but her next comments suggested the lecture was over.

"OK she said. I want to see you in one month, and *during* that time I want you to drink NO alcohol, eat NO carbohydrates, dairy products, fatty meats etc, and then come back and see me."

"I am going to back to Tenerife next week" I said, and have to come back on February 24th which is 6 weeks away, will it be a problem if I make an appointment to see you on the 25th ?"

"No, that just means two more weeks of behaving yourself. Get your self a blood test a few days before you leave

Tenerife and bring the result back to me". She scribbled out a blood test form listing all the tests that were required. She handed it to me saying "I will see you at 11.30 on February 25th....Goodbye" She didn't get up, she didn't open the door for me, but I felt that I was leaving the company of a lady, who, however scary, really knew her business. As I closed the door he final remarks drifted out to me.

"White fish, Salad and spa water is good"

Since I had discovered that being googled was not some form of arcane sexual deviation, I had googled daily. Accordingly, as soon as I reached the privacy of my own home, I set about some specific googling. The keywords LIVER, PCO, and DAMAGE featured large

CHAPTER 12

HAVE A HEART

Tina Wagner was next on my list of hurdles to be overcome. Tina was described in the letter she had written to me as *The Cardio Vascular Nurse* it appeared that she wanted me to walk, and then run upon a treadmill whilst having various leads attached to my person. I felt quite relaxed about this.

I arrived at the hospital in fine fettle. I eventually found my way to the appropriate department and gave my name to reception. "Please take a seat over there" said the receptionist without giving me any indication as to where 'there' might be. So I asked her.

"Where's there?'" I said.

"There's 'there'" she answered, giving a vague nod of her head towards an area occupied by several thousand people some gowned and some un-gowned. I made my way over to an area where the majority of the waiting throngs were in 'mufti'

"Basil Jay" said a voice, I looked around, a muscular young man in white trousers, a white tee shirt and a flapping white coat, was standing by an open door which bore the legend *'cardio vascular' dept.'*

"Tina?" I enquired interrogatively.

"No" he answered monosybalically

"A joke" I ventured apologetically

"Come through" he replied his face breaking into a grin as he said "Tina's off today…..and anyway she has bigger muscles. The ice was broken.

The room was very small. Along the window wall, which looked out over the hospital dustbins, was a treadmill of the kind found in any self respecting gym. Next to the treadmill was a small desk with a computer and large printer which had several hundred leads coming from it. Next to the desk was a very tall, gangling, middle aged, mustachioed, black gentleman who looked exceedingly unhappy…almost morose.

"No", he beat me to the draw, I 'm not Tina either". He gave me a broad grin which showed startling white teeth like new ma jong tiles.

"I wasn't looking for Tina **Either**" I said, taking a chance and purposely mis-understanding, I was told to report to Tina *Wagner*"

"I'm Doctor Rhamatt", he said without moving the grin, "and I am going to have to do"

"You're going to have to do what?" I asked, feeling that I had two companions willing to lighten my medical day. He was prepared to play the game.

"I am going to have to decide whether it is advisable for you spend your money on a season ticket" he said "so let's get on with it shall we". He turned to the young muscular man, and in a voice reminiscent of Captain Kirk of Starship Enterprise saying 'Beam me up Scotty', said with a drawl. "Wire him up Gavin"

Gavin told me to take the chair that stood next to the treadmill and to remove my shirt. After my consultation with Dr. YY Lypin I was a little embarrassed by my Prominent Central Obesity, but I did as I was told, sucking my cheeks, and by definition my PCO in at the same time.

"You can relax" said Gavin; "I'm in a serious relationship". He then draped a dozen cables over his arm before further draping them over the hand-rail of the treadmill, and unsheathed a small brightly coloured razor. 'Lady Shave' I read the words on the box from which the razor had appeared.

"I am just going to remove some of your chest hair" he said, "so that I can get better adhesion with the contacts". Although I had grown as attached to my chest hair as it had grown attached to me, I watched its departure with hardly a tear, knowing that it was nothing that a few months of patient nurturing wouldn't once more replenish in all their bushless glory. Eventually he declared himself satisfied and proceeded to attach the contact points to the bare areas, before retrieving the cables from the treadmill and clipping them in place. The gangling Dr Rhamhatt said nothing, but continued to quietly gangle whilst he waited for his day to improve.

"OK" said Gavin, "we are all set, and so I will tell you what I want you to do…first, stand up and move onto the treadmill". I stood up and moved onto the treadmill. "Have you ever been on one before?" he asked

"Many times at the gym" I answered

"Good" he said, "so you know what to do." I nodded. "The only difference is that you are now attached to the computer which will read the re-action of your heart as we take you through the various levels. There will be a lot of clattering as the machine prints out its log, but I don't want you to worry about that, you just keep on walking"

"Like Felix" I said,

"Who?" he looked quizzical

"Oh, just a comic book character of a long time ago" I said, he didn't ask for further details, but simply carried on with his instructions.

"Just breathe normally and each two or three minutes I will increase the speed. If you suffer any discomfort at all, just tell me and I will stop the machine" He looked at me, "Are you OK with that?"

"Absolutely", I said, "Lead on McDuff"

"I suppose he's a friend of Felix" he said as he pressed the button.

I must say I found it all rather straight forward .... at first. We went through level one – the only pants in sight were the top of my yellow Y fronts, where my trousers had slipped down my hips. Level 2 was OK, but I didn't feel like bursting into song. Level three began to give me a bit of problem, but not one I was prepared to admit to, and when Gavin asked if I was OK, I simply nodded so that he would not be aware that I needed every bit of oxygen available for the simple process of staying upright. But he guessed.

"I would like to try one more level" he said "are you OK with that?" I nodded in time with my heart beat. The speed now seemed equivalent to that at which Roger Bannister made history in the fifties over the magic mile. I could no longer suppress the heavy breathing, and for the first time, Dr R. began to ungangle himself and look closely at the ECG read-out, allowing the paper to thread through his fingers.

"Are you OK?" said Gavin, "just two more minutes, can you manage that?"

"Yes" I breathed with my next exhalation, as long as it's no more. Gavin began to help

"90 seconds, 75 seconds, one minute" it wasn't helping, I was just concentrating on making my feet keep up with the speed of the floor I was trying to stand on. "45 seconds, 30 seconds" I could taste success, I knew I would complete the test whilst still standing upright. "15 seconds". I remembered the treadmill in the gym, where, at the end of the programme one went through a cooling down period where the floor slowed down significantly, but did not come to an immediate stop. I prepared for it and was confident that my feet would remember how to go slower. "10, 9, 8, 7, 6, 5, 4, 3, 2, 1 OK, hit the button", this latter instruction to the gangling Dr. Rhamatt. The next thing I remember was the floor moving noticeably faster and me looking up at Gavin from the kneeling position.

"Sorry" said Dr Rhamatt. Luckily as I went to my knees, Gavin had simultaneously pulled the emergency switch, and no damage had been done. "Whoops" said gangling Dr Rhamatt, as I pulled myself to my feet.

"Ouch" said exhausted Basil Jay

"Sh*t" said muscular Gavin. I was just grateful that he had pulled the emergency switch which had stopped the treadmill dead, thus preventing me from ending up the same way.

"There, that wasn't so bad, was it?" said the gangling Dr Rhamatt.

"sorry about that" said Gavin as he disconnected me from the machine and tore of the adhesive contacts and whatever hair he had failed to shave off the first time. "You can put your shirt on now". With trembling hands I buttoned up my shirt and tucked my PCO into my trousers before sitting heavily on the chair.

"I will send the report to your GP" said Dr Rhamatt, but I can tell you that you haven't got angina"

I was grateful to the doctor for telling me what I hadn't got, and realized that I would have to wait for the lovely Nita to tell me what I had got. But for now I had had enough, and was ready to head for home a good stiff tomato juice.

CHAPTER 13

A FLASHBACK TO THE BS4B- 1

I sipped my good stiff tomato juice, having been **persuaded** by Scary Lady to go **mega**-easy on the vodka. I did as I was told, and, as always happens to a dying *(for a drink)* man, my past life played out before me. I closed my eyes and let it play. Suddenly I was back in the good old days, when my only medical problem was a, probably incurable, overactive tongue.

I want to tell you about one of my favourite bank managers, Terry Halibut….No of course that isn't his real name, let's face it, to have a doctor called Nita Hakelin and a bank manager named Terry Halibut would be ….well… just too fishy for words.

Terry would, by now, be a young man in his early nineties with his whole future banking career stretching out behind him, and how unfair of me would it be to put that at risk.

I've just told one of my little fibs again….the fact is that Terry retired from the bank just at the time that I was contemplating the Isle of Man. I was 48 and he would have been just a little over 50. Somebody once said of my partner Ken and I. "You two are becoming quite a commercial force in this town." I can't re-call who said it, but it was probably me. Anyway, Terry Halibut followed a short though eminent procession of bank managers who had been our support during the early years of the 1980's. Magic years when to borrow a million pounds from a bank all you had to do was manage to walk as far as the bank managers office without tripping over your shoelaces *(which is why I wear slip-ons to this very day)*. It was made easier by the fact that to make money in the property business you had to fully understand the market. However, that understanding seldom needed to project beyond knowing that…Buying on Monday and selling on Tuesday usually resulted in a profit most satisfactory.

But what about these bank managers, bless 'em. First we had Frank…not so much a 'given' name as one resulting from his endearing habit of leaning with both elbows on his desk, fixing you with a myopic stare, and saying….."I'm going to be FRANK with you. I think his real name was Gerry, but he seemed quite happy to fit into our little world. Next there came PEERBOB. Now then, this name came about by accident. On his taking over the branch, Ken and I, as we always did, were amongst the first to offer him a free lunch and tell him who he should nuzzle up to and who he should avoid in our small town business hierarchy. Well being, as somebody had clearly told him, a 'commercial force in the town' *(that was probably me as well)* he accepted our invitation with alacrity *(No not Franks old secretary who was still hanging on for her pension whilst running the bank whilst her bosses were out to lunch – her name was, and probably still is, Verity)*. The new man's name was Mr. Pearson, and, being good clients we collected him from the bank on the given day, bundled him into Ken's Range Rover, and set of for the local Hotel which boasted the best restaurant in the town together with tables set amongst fake palm trees and rubber plants behind which one could easily hide if passing a little brown envelope ever became an issue.

"Hello Mr. Pearson" I began, whilst Ken was busy grinding his gears, as well as his teeth. Ken wasn't really in favour in lunching with people he didn't know just for the sake of PR. "Welcome to our town.....I am sure we are going to have a very good relationship" He merely nodded, oh dear, was he cast in Ken's mould I wondered. Our short journey to the Hotel was made in comparative silence, even though I tried to break the ice by saying. "I'm Basil and this is Ken, by the way". This important bit of information was received with a curt nod and no indication as to whether or not he had a first name with which we were to come to terms. Ken parked outside the Hotel, the sun was shining, the sea was strangely blue, and I could see, there stretched before me, the prospect of one and a half hours of oral hardship as I tried to keep a conversation flowing between myself and two men who clearly didn't want to be there. There was a minor breakthrough as we climbed out of the car.

"I'm Bob" Mr. Pearson said, just that, and he strode off to Hotel's front entrance with Ken and I shrugging and bringing up the rear. His name was carved in stone within seconds of our sitting down. Ken decided he must offer something.

"Well Mr. Peer......" he started, and then remembered the first name olive branch and with a near seamless transition added "Bob" Of course, what came out was "Well Mr. Peerbob" The die was cast and it was an opportunity I simply could not pass up.

"You don't mind us calling you Peerbob.....do you?" I asked with a grin, we do have pet names for all our *'favourite'* (*a word I clearly spoke in italics as opposed to Esperanto*) The man was human. His face cracked into a big grin, he beamed at us both and said.

"Not at all, in fact, I think I am going to like it here".

Peerbob, Ken and I became firm friends, sadly brought to an end when he was promoted to a bigger job, in a bigger branch, in a bigger town, for a bigger salary. As Ken remarked

"What a bugger he prefers bigger".

But of course I do not want to talk to you about Frank, or even Peerbob, but about his successor, Terry Halibut. Now where Peerbob was confident of his skills and his authority, Terry always gave the impression that he was a little bit in awe of what he had achieved. One thing we had established with Peerbob was a fairly health 'credit line' which meant we didn't have to 'prove' every deal to the bank, although we always gave them a cash flow projection on when we would need draw-downs, etc. etc. Peerbob had been very relaxed about this, as, I have to say, what anyone in business in the eighties will tell, it was a time when most bank managers did 'relaxed'. The oft used words were "we lend to the man, NOT the project" had dropped from many a bank managers lips during that magic period when bank managers tended to wear long trousers…. oh happy days. Anyway, to continue, Terry was clearly a nervous man, and although he did not suggest any amendment to our arrangement, he did ask us to go in on one occasion soon after his induction lunch at the Cooden Beach Hotel, and flesh out one of our proposals. I prepared a fairly lengthy outline of the project, which essentially entailed buying an old cinema and bingo hall with an attached printing works *(in a high street position, the printers having moved out to a modern business park)* and creating a small, but much needed shopping mall with offices over. Ken and I sat the other side of Terry's desk and, each of us with a copy of project details, began to skim through it. Skim, sadly enough, was not a word in Terry's vocabulary. After perhaps twenty minutes of him dissecting every sentence and asking for explanations on numerous figures Ken banged, gently, on his desk.

"Look Terry he said" and fixed him with his cheeky gap toothed smile *(before he became my partner he used to be a professional footballer with a well known London club)* which belied the hard glint in his eye. "We buy it for this"…. He tapped the paper firmly with his finger. "We spend this on the building work and fees". Another pronounced tapping. "And we sell it for this" another seriously macho tap on the paper. "The difference is the profit, and this is it". He now plonked a fist down on the bottom line. "Now then, are you going to lend us the F**ing money or not?"

"When do you need your first draw down?" said Terry. But I was the nice guy and it was clearly time for me to intercede.

"Wait a minute Ken, fair's fair," I said, "Terry has got to make sure that he is covering all the bases and he needs to fully understand the deal" Ken said nothing, he had seen me in this conciliatory mode before and probably guessed that I had a compromise to suggest. I went on, this time to Terry.

"Terry, I know exactly what you need. Every month for our internal use" *(no I wasn't getting medical)*, I produce a set of figures, they are updated by the computer every 28 days and it sets out ALL the projects that are on-going, showing interim positions, budget analysis and monthly summaries. It is our 'Form BS4B-1. Provided our accountant has no objections I will make sure a confidential copy is sent to you every month…will that help?" The resulting beaming face was a picture.

"Basil, that will be marvelous, it will keep my files up

to date and help with any embarrassing questions I may be asked" We shook hands and left the bank. As we strolled back to our office Ken turned to me and said

"What the F**K is a BS4B-1?"

"No idea", I said, "but I expect I can come up with something."

Terry was our manager for almost three years, and we did big things together. Each month I would religiously send him this complicated spreadsheet which he duly filed without once, in the whole of relationship asking any questions about it. His retirement really co-incided with Ken and I deciding we were ready to throw in the towel as well. We took Terry to the Cooden Beach for a final 'business lunch', and after a very pleasant hour or three, Terry said

"I'll miss you two buggers" he smiled, "but I certainly won't miss your monthly BS4B's" he went on "It must have been a bit of a bastard having to update that every month when it was of no practical use to man nor beast"

"What do you mean?" I said, "beginning to get an inkling of what he meant"

"When I got the first one, I was truly smitten with its depth and detail, BUT, by the third I was beginning to wonder about them. I began to wonder 'why the document should be named a BS4B, none of the initials were familiar to me in either accounting terms, or within your own company's names. Then it hit me BS4B. **B**ull **S**hit **4 B**anks. I worked that out after the third. He reached down under the table and pulled up a soft document case, he withdrew a file and placed in front of me. You went on to produce 29 more, each of which, I quietly placed in the file without reading and longing for this day". He beamed around the table at us, and Ken and l saw the funny side of it. Before long we were all laughing out loud. Terry brought us back to earth.

"Just be thankful that nothing went wrong with any of your deals, because if it had of done, I would have had you by the balls."

Here's to you Terry Halibut....where-ever you are, you have been a part of Basil's wonderful journey. Thank you

Chapter 14

HE'S A BRAVE LITTLE SOLDIER

After that little detour, let's get back to internal strife of Basil Jay.

In July I was first given the opportunity to impress the world 'again' by being, as my dear old mum always told me, a 'brave little soldier'. It happened when I attended the appointment with the doctor to whom The Lovely Nita had decided I should pay 'LIP' service. I have to say, that of all the bits dropping off, or threatening to drop off in the years since 2004, the sunburned lip problem, although refusing to go away, worried me the least. That was until I met Doctor Michael Alonso. Clearly, I thought, a throwback from the Spanish Inquisition. An improbable and silly thought, which, soon seemed to become, less silly and less improbable.

I had to attend his clinic, courtesy of my insurance company. He collected me from the waiting room. "Welcome Mr. Jay ... Basil", at that time I did not notice his two incisors rubbing against the point of his chin. "Now" he said, according to this letter from......" he paused and turned over the page... "Dr. Hakelin, you have had a sunburned lip since your sojourn" *(did people still use words like this)* "in the wonderful Canaries – where" he added with a chuckle " Lord Nelson lost his eye"

"His arm" I said

"No, I think you will find it was his eye" he replied. I was right, Nelson lost his arm in the Battle of Santa Cruz in 1797, but who cares as long as our gallant sailor had not got sunburned lips, and anyway, one does not contradict a know it all Doctor to whom you owe enough lip to take a biopsy. So I just smiled apologetically at my ignorance.

"Yes, his eye" he said almost at a whisper before saying, "Now let me look at this lip" he pouted in case I was not sure what a lip was. I proved my knowledge of human anatomy by pouting back.

"Ahhhhh" he said, and I suddenly realized he had been to the same medical school as Mr. Breading, so I was able to respond – through pouting lips.

"Ummmmmmm"

"Nasty" he said, "I will need to take a sample for the lab, it will take but a jiffy"

"Good Lord" I thought, he's got a jiffy as well. It must be some sort of hospital conveyance. He went, I stayed, a nurse patted my hand

"It will only take a moment" she said, "and you won't feel a thing". Meaning….this will take a while, and it will hurt like hell. It did, and it did. Dr. Alonso produced this little gadget that looked like the kitchen implement used for taking cores out of apples. "Here we go" said Dr. A, it is very quick and you won't need an anesthetic." Meaning…. sorry chum, rather you than me without an anesthetic, but sadly the anesthetist is on his tea break. He placed the implement against my lip and pressed. "BLOODY ADA", I cried out through pouted top lip….. because from the level of the pain, I had no doubt that he had just carved away the whole of my bottom lip.

"There" he said, "that wasn't so bad was it". I couldn't answer because I was too busy trying to stop the blood dripping onto my white shirt.

"I will send this off to lab for a biopsy" he said, and then send the result to your GP". With that, he stalked out of the door, and I, for one, was not sorry to see him go.

I reflected. It was August, 2008, ironically almost exactly 4 years since I was first diagnosed with galloping prostate cancer. Since then, despite having had my prostate removed, the cancer had returned twice. I have enjoyed a period, as relayed earlier in this book of Hormone Therapy and Radio Therapy, which seemed to have sorted the matter out. But, in February of 2008 my PSA had begun to rise again. At a consultation with my dear friend and Doctor Henry Draper, he fingered my blood test report, steepled his fingers, tried to look very earnest – which isn't easy if your name is Henry, and to my question "How am I Doctor?" he said.

"It's disappointing. It's *very* disappointing. Since December, your PSA has reason from 0.1 to 0.4. Not high in itself, but growing at a rate which is very disappointing" He sighed, before repeating "Yes…*very* disappointing" He looked so sad, I was tempted to put my arm around him and say,

"There there 'old man' don't let it get you down." Instead, I said "well, what do you recommend?"

"Let's not panic" he said, and I had visions of Corporal Jones from Dad's Army rushing around the surgery with his famous line……..Don't panic, don't panic Mr. Mainwaring. He went on. "Let's have another look in a couple of months and see what is happening. We have a sort of 'rule of thumb', and if the level doubles over less than 8 months we like to look seriously at the problem" Did he mean that up to now it had all been a bit of 'knock about' fun' I wondered. Anyway, he pulled himself together, let out another sigh, un-steepled his fingers, stood up with a smile and said. "When are you going back to Tenerife?"

"Within a couple of days I said"

"When are you back?" he asked

""End of April or beginning of May" Polly answered

"But earlier if needs be" I added.

"Why don't you get a blood test in Tenerife towards the end of March, and we will see how things are going". It seemed that a decision had been made, and with a quip on my sadly depleted lips, a spring in my step, and a nasty lump in the pit of my stomach, I bade him farewell.

I was, of course, now well under the control of Scary Lady, by this time about a stone lighter than the day I had met her, and feeling pretty good.

My treatment at the hands of the Spanish Inquisition had appeared to yield no real problem, and an English summer stretched ahead of me with no more than rain, high winds, and possibly a depression over Kent

to spoil my enjoyment.

It was to stay that way for a month or two, until we discovered that my PSA had not only doubled in less than eight months (five to be precise) BUT had climbed to 1.1, an increase by a factor of almost three…."Ouch", I said to Polly "Dr Henry will be *VERY* disappointed. And he was……."

"We don't usually worry until it reaches double figures" he said at our next consultation.

"Explain to me" I asked, exactly what is happening…… and then, before he could utter a word I told him what I thought was happening.

"As I see it" I said, "when Mr. Breading removed my prostate he left behind a small amount of tissue, which, gradually started to obtain a cancerous growth". Dr. Draper nodded sagely, "Last year you were concerned about the rapid growth as indicated by my PSA. It went, you will recall", he allowed himself to re-call. "from 0.1 to 0.7 in around four months". He nodded. "When it reached 0.7 you asked for an MRI scan, and a full body scan". He nodded again. "You then put me on a course of hormone therapy and after the MRI results which identified the cancer in the prostate bed you put me on four weeks of daily radiation therapy". His nodding was now so prolonged that there was a danger of his head coming loose and landing on top of his steepled fingers. I paused to take a breath before finishing "If so much was necessary with a PSA of 0.7, why now are you recommending that we 'wait and see' when it is 1.1". His nodding got markedly slower, all danger of a 'bouncing bonce' immediately receded and smile lit up his face.

"Let me try to explain" he said. I let him try to explain, but said

"I'll try to understand" I gave him a grin to show him it was meant light-heartedly.

"When we use radiation we not only kill the cancer, but there is always a danger that we will harm healthy tissue". It was my turn to nod. "Your MRI and body scans both showed that the cancer was not present in the bones, nor in the lymph nodes", by way of explanation he explained that these were the normal areas to which prostate cancer was prone to spread. He continued. "Neither he said, has it spread to any of the surrounding tissue or organs". He paused to make sure I was really understanding. I pulled an 'I'm really understanding' sort of a face. He carried on, clearly pleased that I was keeping up. "Now, although it is very disappointing that your PSA is once again on the rise, it is very doubtful that there will be any 'treatable' evidence of it until your PSA gets into double figures. In fact it is not unusual *after* a radical prostatectomy to see PSA levels rise to as much as 40". He paused to allow it to sink in. I allowed it to sink in.

"Can you arrange for me to have an MRI please?" I said.

"Of course" he said "But not only that, I will put you back on a six month course of hormone therapy, this, as I think I explained last time, effectively *'blocks'* the testosterone, and prevents it reaching the cancer. Prostate cancer feeds of testosterone, and if we starve it, in many cases it simply dies away."

"That's fine" I said, "Last time I put on over 2 stone in weight. This time I will be more aware and monitor my weight with care, having", I couldn't resist adding, "lost between three and a half and four stone since I reached my maximum last year"

"Did you get on OK with the side effects?" he asked

"You mean the *hot flushes* and *sticky out jumpers*", I said "I suppose the answer is yes….and no. The hot flushes I could cope with, the sensitive nipples and 34c cup was a bit more difficult" I went on "and do you know, the irony is that, although I have lost all of this weight, my breasts still rival a young Dolly Parton" I was warming to a theme that I had not intended to raise with him. "In fact, because a strict diet has clearly worked, but failed to reduce the breast area, I have been looking at cosmetic surgery. The problem is called Guy..maaa"

"Gynecomastia" he helped me out

"The procedure is common and simple…usually as an outpatient, but at most an overnighter, and involves liposuction and a very small scar under the nipple"

"You've really investigated this" A voice from the corner, as Polly, who had been listening carefully and saying nothing, had suddenly chipped in.

"Googling must be a nightmare for you doctors" I said to Dr Harry

"Not at all" he said pretending to tap a keyboard on his knee", he smiled…..."How do you think we find out about these things?" we all smiled…..dutifully.

"Anyway" he said, "to wrap things up, I will leave a note with the hospital regarding the MRI scan, and if you give them a ring tomorrow and get a date, and then phone Jo, my secretary, and she will set up an appointment for us to discuss the results – but don't worry about them, with a PSA of 1.1 they will almost certainly be negative"

"Thank you"

"Oh" said Harry "and don't forget to see your GP to get the hormone treatment started".

"I won't" I said, and, glad that we were doing something again, I took my sweater, my umbrella, my wife, and my leave of the 'easy to like' Dr Harry Draper, and walked confidently into the sunset.

The next day was a Friday. First I phoned my local surgery and asked for an appointment with *any* of the Doctors. The lovely Nita was on pregnancy leave and I didn't have a particular affinity with any of the others. An appointment was made for me to see a Dr. Crainer, who was apparently filling in for the lovely Nita during the six months of her pre and post delivery leave. After that I phoned Winterlands. The conversation was interesting.

"Good morning, Winterlands Hospital, Janine speaking"

"Good morning Janine, my name is Basil Jay, and I would like to make an appointment to have an MRI scan"

"Hello Mr. Jay, can I ask who your consultant is?"

"Yes…it is Dr. Harry Draper…I saw him last night….. he was going to leave a note with you"

"Ah! That would have gone to X-Ray…I'll just 'pop' you through"

"Thank you Janine"

"XRAY"

"Good morning, my name is Basil Jay"

"Ah yes…good morning Mr. Jay, I have Dr Drapers note in front of me….would 11.0 Sunday morning be convenient?"

"That's the day after tomorrow"

"That's right"

"I didn't expect it to be so quick"

"Well it's a mobile unit and visits us Tuesdays and Sundays….would Tuesday be better?"

"No not at all, Sunday is fine"

"Goooooood, I just have to ask you a few questions"

"Can you confirm your date of birth?"

"Yes"

"And it is"

"28th July 1942"

"Can you give me the first line of your address?" I'd got the hang of it now, so I gave it to her.

"Do you have any metal in your body?"

"Only a Backbone of Steel protecting a Heart of Gold" I said

"Can I take that as a NO then?" laughed X-Ray

"Yes, I did have pins in my feet, but they've been removed"

"That's OK then"

"Oh wait a minute….I have some dental implants…. do they count"

"No they will be fine….have you had any surgery in the last three months?"

"No"

"Are you on any medication?"

146

"I gave her the list"

"That's fine then….I'll see you on Sunday…..take care"

"And you…goodbye"

So that was pretty easy. Next stop Dr Crainer.

BASIL JAY TO ROOM 9

I just love these automated gadgets, not quite as much fun as the old days, when the *'outgoing'* patient would say NEXT in the general direction of the waiting hoards. I went to room 9. I expected Dr Crainer to be wearing short trousers and sucking a lollipop. But no. Dr Crainer was probably in his early forties, very affable and exuding a comforting aura of competence.

"Good morning Mr. Jay" he said "How can I help you this morning?" I told him of my appointment with Dr Harry and that he was writing to explain the medication to be prescribed.

"If it was only yesterday I doubt if it is on the computer yet" he said

"I thought that was a possibility I said, but Dr Draper emailed me after our appointment with the details". I had printed off the email and handed it to him.

"This is unusual" he said, "I am not sure I will be able to prescribe on the strength of an email". He tapped on his keyboard. "Well fancy that" he said, "the letter is here, together with a copy of one to Mr. Breading"

"He was the surgeon who operated" I explained

"Just let me read it" he said pleasantly, and then "Yes that's fine, Dr Draper is recommending intermittent hormone therapy, six months on and six months off"

"Is he" I said, quite sure that he had never mentioned that part to me, and slightly concerned that my breasts would be inflating and deflating like balloons at a fair.

"Easy done" said Dr Crainer, and printed me out the prescription. "Anything else I can do for you?" he said

"Well" I responded, I have an MRI scan on Sunday"

"On Sunday"

"On Sunday"

"When was this arranged?"

"Yesterday"

"Yesterday?"

"Yes, Yesterday"

"It must be private"

"Yes it is….courtesy of the SL insurance company, who, I must say have been brilliant over the last 4 years"

"Private Medicine is a wonderful thing". I got the feeling his whole heart wasn't behind the statement. "On the NHS you would have no chance of an MRI scan with a PSA reading of just 1.1. It would need to be well into double figures, and then you would have to wait a lot longer than *two days*". He emphasized the time element.

"I consider myself very fortunate" I said, and I must say, I too feel the imbalance between private medicine and the NHS is outrageous" He seemed encouraged by my response.

"Is everything else OK?" he asked

"Well, no" I said. "For the past three months or so I have had a very dry throat, with a tickling dry cough which recurs every half hour or so and makes it difficult for me to talk. It only lasts for, perhaps, five minutes". I paused, not wanting to say the next bit, but I rushed on. "I have a problem at the moment, knowing that there is unattached and growing cancer tissue floating around looking for somewhere to land, every time I get a pain in my toe, or a lump on my knee, or……a dry tickling cough, I assume the worst, and that", I searched my memory for a suitable simile, I found one and

quote from one of my favourite Jack Higgins books "that…
the eagle has landed" I finished.

Dr Crainer appeared not to be listening; he was busy
tapping on his computer. Having come this far I carried on
regardless. "Ironically a good friend of mine was diagnosed
a couple of weeks ago with cancer of the oesophagus
and…………" I let the sentence trail away, expecting him
to say….'For God's sake man….pull your-self together'. He
didn't.

"Your worry is quite understandable, but let me put your
mind a rest. I have just been going through your records
on the computer"; and here's me thinking he was playing
solitaire until I had left the room. "I see you were prescribed
Ramipril earlier this year"

"Yes, I offered, "highish blood pressure"

"Did you read the leaflet that comes in the box?"

"No"

"Tut, double tut" but said with a smile. "I quote…
'Ramipril may cause a dry cough and tickling in the throat.
If persistent consult your Doctor'" He smiled "So, you see,
you have done absolutely the right thing. I will change your
tablets, but first I think I'll give you a good examination.
Take your shirt off please"

Wow, suddenly I was being treated like a proper patient;
my early impression of competence was being borne out.
The examination was thorough and at the end he said "Well
everything sounds fine. Your blood pressure is up but that is
probable because of the surgery environment"

"I take my blood pressure every morning, by order of Dr
YY Lypin, I said, this morning it was 128 over 83, which in
itself is higher than usual"

"Tell you what I would like you to do then…here is your
new prescription to replace the Ramipril. I am putting you
on Cozaar. Make an appointment to come and see my again

in four weeks and bring with you your own blood pressure readings. By then your tickly throat should be a thing of the past". I reached out and took the prescription from him.

"Thank you Doctor……very much" I stood up to go

"Don't forget your hormones he said, picking the prescription from of his desk"

"I'll see you in a month" I said…smiling. As I reached the door he said

"Mr. Jay", I turned

"Yes Doctor"

"The usual symptom for cancer of the oesophagus is difficulty in swallowing, so don't worry any more about your dry cough"

When I got home I studied my new hormone tablets BICALUTAMIDE. I read the leaflet. The side effects were listed under:-

In more than one in ten patients
In fewer than one in ten patients
In fewer than one in one hundred patients
In fewer than one in one thousand patients
In fewer than one in ten thousand patients

There were a total of TWENTY SEVEN side effects. With the worst, under the final category. LIVER FAILURE, But the one that I found ironic, was under the one in one hundred category. Can cause a TICKLY THROAT AND DRY COUGH.

Sunday morning at slightly before 11am I presented myself at the reception of Winterlands.

"Good Morning, I am Basil Jay; I spoke to you on Friday". It was, indeed, Janine.

"Good morning Janine, I am a little early"

"That's fine," she answered, "they are actually ready for you now, I'll just phone through"

An Asian gentleman in his thirties responded to the phone call in seconds and appeared before me.

"Good morning Mr. Jay" he said, "if you are ready we can get started"

"Perhaps a quick visit to the loo first" I asked

"Of course" he said "do you know where it is?"

"Does the Pope wear a funny hat?" I said, realizing he may not know whether he does or not, I thought about the bear in the woods, but then thought, perhaps not. Instead I expanded upon my Pope simile, "When you have had a radical prostatectomy the location of the loos in every building you ever visit becomes your first priority. Besides, over the past four years I have spent a fair amount of time in this particular building" I noticed that Janine was struggling unsuccessfully to keep a straight face. After the loo stop I returned to reception saying.

"Lead on McDuff". My new young friend led on.

The mobile scanning unit was in the car-park and approached up a steepish set of stairs. I negotiated my way to the top without difficulty and sat in the chair indicated by another young man who could have been my guide's brother.

"Hello Mr. Jay" he said, "have you had an MRI scan before?"

"This will be my third" I replied

"Before we start" he said, "I need to ask you a few questions" he then proceeded to ask the same questions that I had answered on Friday. I was as good as gold, made no smart alec responses, and the matter took no more than a couple of minutes. "This scan will last about 50 minutes", he said. He fingered my wrist watch. "Is the watch gold" he said, at first I thought he was going to make me an offer, but he quickly went on "MRI stands for Magnetic Resonance Imaging, by definition magnets re-act to metal" He smiled, a big toothy smile, it does NOT re-act gold". We had a quick inventory, neck chain, rings etc. "Now Mr. Jay, if you would like to pop through that door and slip on one of the gowns we can get started". I 'popped' through the door and 'slipped' into a gown that came just about level with the top of my thighs. I guessed there would be some trousers somewhere, but there weren't. I 'popped' back through the door to be greeted by

"Mr. Jay, could you not find any bottoms". He ushered me back through the door and found me some bottoms in a cupboard. I slipped them on and was ready to go.

If you have not had an MRI scan, leave your claustrophobia at home. You lie on a table that then slides into a very tight and very low tunnel. Your nose is inches from the top and your arms tight to your sides with your hands folded on your chest. The perfect position for the undertaker if you happen to croak mid way. My new best friend gave me a panic button with the instruction if you have any problems at all just 'press' this button and we will have you out of here as soon as......we have finished our tea break'. No he didn't say that at all, he said "in seconds".

The process of the scan was uneventful. I heard some early giggling, but eventually dozed off. I later found that the giggling was probably caused by the fact that, some months previously, deciding I was probably old enough, Polly had allowed to go out and buy my own socks. I had bought SEVEN pairs, each pair had, across the sole, the 'day of the week' in big letters. On the day of my scan I had put on a 'pair', the right foot of which said Tuesday, whilst my left foot proclaimed it to be Friday. Lying, as I was, on my back in the scanner my legs were elevated giving my two operatives a enhanced view of my feet. Into every life one tries to bring a little sunshine.

On Thursday at 6.pm. Polly and I arrived at Winterlands for an appraisal of my MRI scan which Dr Harry had assured me would show nothing. A bad omen occurred as I was parking the car. The self selector lever snapped off and the car was stuck in Drive. I had parked with the nose pressed tight to the wall and so the only way out was to reverse. I decided to worry about it later but was convinced that I could steer it successfully so long as Polly put her back into it and pushed me backwards. I signed in and the lady on reception recorded my presence. We took a seat in the comfortable waiting room. We were fifteen minutes early, and I was about to get myself a cappuccino when Dr Harry walked in to the waiting room and said

"Ready." I was as ready as I would be likely to be although we had discussed what would come out of the consultation and Polly had said

"Simple, he will say that nothing is showing and come and see him in three months" Hey Ho, Hey Ho. He opened the door and we went in, he indicated two chairs and we sat down – one of us in each. He sat behind his desk and did his 'steepling fingers' bit. I knew we were in trouble by his opening line

"I have some good news" It was not a level statement I-HAVE-SOME-GOOD-NEWS. Oh no! it was delivered with the intonation which tells you I have some good news AND. And so it was.

"The scan shows that the bones and the organs and the Lymph Nodes are clear BUT..........in the prostate bed itself there is clearly defined an area of about 6mm by 4mm which is cancerous tissue.....It is surprising......It is **very** surprising",

He went further "in countless patients you are the only one that has shown such a phenomenon"

"Oh dear" I said. "What do we do?"

"Well, our options are rather limited" He paused and fell into his familiar pose of the steepled fingers. He unclasped his hands in order to give himself some spare fingers to count with.

"One" he said holding up a solitary digit, "we can't give you any more radiation therapy because we have bombarded the prostate bed daily for four consecutive weeks, and, well frankly, I don't think it could take any more" He shrugged. "Two", he held up another digit, "we can do what we are doing, namely let oestrogen do the work for us by blocking the entrance to the prostate bed and denying the cancer the testosterone it needs to feed on and grow....I have to say that that is not a one hundred percent certainty however". "Three", where does he get all these fingers from, "we can move into the realms of advanced experimentation". He stopped talking and looked at me.

"What are you suggesting?" I asked

"Have you ever heard of CryoblationTherapy?" he asked

"Ouch" I said, "I have heard of Cryogentics where the wealthy with incurable diseases have themselves frozen for one hundred years in the hope that when they are brought back to life a cure will have been found for whatever ails them". He gave a little chuckle,

"you're on the right lines he said, but cryoblation, or cryo-therapy is no where near so drastic as that"

"Well", I said "even 50 years will put Polly slightly past her prime"

"Not even 50 years" he said. "Here we are talking about cryo-surgery, where a probe is entered into your body, and directed at the source of the cancer, it is then subjected to a blast of Nitrogen which is 50 degrees below freezing. The cold kills the cancer"

"Not too good for brass monkeys then", I said trying to keep the mood light.

"No, but potentially very good news for you". Good answer I thought.

"We don't do it in Maidstone, he said, the nearest hospital is at Tunbridge Wells, the surgeon, and a major innovator in prostate cancer cures, is Professor Hardly, and, with your permission I would like to write to him, send him all your scans, and ask him to give you a consultation". He gave me one of his serious looks before continuing, "It will be his decision whether the treatment is appropriate in your case.

"Permission granted" I said.

"I will write tomorrow" he said "I have to get all of these" he hafted the thick envelope of my scans "over to him, but I will try to set it up as quickly as I can" He paused "Are you around for long?"

"Doesn't that depend on the success of the treatment" I said, and then relenting said, "pretty much to the end of September, BUT, I do have ten days golf in Ireland from the 8th".

"We'll try to work around those dates" he said. I shook his hand and Polly and I started towards the door. "Basil" he said,

"Yes", which seemed an appropriate reply

"Did you mention that your car is in the car park stuck in Drive and with no reverse" he said in an *'I'd love to help you if I could'* sort of voice.

"I did" I replied, in an *'Aren't I a silly billy then'* kind of a voice whilst welcoming his interest and upcoming help.

"I hope you're not blocking me in" he said with a grin.

There is no doubt about it, being ill is not all alarm and despondency.

Polly put her back into it, I wrestled the gear into neutral and steered very professionally backwards, whilst Polly dug her toes into the moist August ground and pushed like a good'un. Deed done we set of for an early dinner at Kits Coty, in the top three of our favourite restaurants.

In Kent. I did the driving. It was, I felt, the very least I could do.

CHAPTER 15

HERE COME THE TIGERS

At the moment I am living in a curious 'Half Asleep' world. That IS to say, I am 'Half Asleep' during the day when I should be 'Wide Awake', and I am 'Wide Awake' in the middle of the night when I should be slightly more than 'Half Asleep'

I drink too much! Now I don't want you to infer from that, that I am in training to join AA, or even the RAC, neither do I suggest that I am 'oft inebriated'. I neither want, nor need a couple of vodkas with my breakfast cereal. On golfing days I happily allow my water bottle to contain ordinary water as opposed to firewater. If I am otherwise constructively employed, cups of coffee more than fill the beverage gap. But, when not golfing, the simple fact is that I like good lunches, and a good lunch, by popular *(as opposed to 'scary lady' definition)* includes a couple of glasses of good wine. And then in the evening Polly and I will share a bottle of Chablis – straight down the middle – one third for her and two thirds for me, and when the bottle is empty I often have an extra glass.

The only spirit I drink is a long Gin and Tonic with

bundles of ice and a slice of lemon. I don't get maudling as the evening progresses. What I do get very introspective. Why do I have those extra couple of glasses each night? I'll tell you, it is in the hope that they will be sufficient to STOP my Tigers coming in the pre-dawn. But they seldom do. I have fortunately inherited or developed an attitude of easy going 'devil take the hindmost' so that my friends and family think it remarkable that I always appear completely happy with my lot – and completely happy with my lot I am. The cheerful grin, the badly told joke. The sense of seeing the best of every situation. All of these things have always come easily to me in the company of friends or family. BUT, we all, every one of us, have our demons. The fact is that over the past few years, I have spent so much pre-dawn time with mine, that they are almost my friends. Friends it must be said, that I am still happy to hold at arms length. There are, however days when I fail, and at 4 o'clock in the morning, when the world is asleep, my Tigers still come...... They remind me of illness.....of pain.... and most of all......of.... of what? Perhaps of not being around anymore, perhaps of missing what, I am sure will be a very special 15 years or so of my life. Perhaps...............OK, so what has brought on all this 'under the surface' self-pity to trouble me anew? I'll tell you.

For some months my Tigers had dwelt at the furthest extremities of my mind, but then, they started to re-visit me again soon after my PSA began to raise fears of cancer's return. At first they were just vaguely taunting.

Fear *was back again with his noisy roaring. "Only one things going to get you free of this returning cancer, Basil me old mate, and you know what that is don't you". He didn't give me a chance to form a reply in my head before rushing on with. "Anyway, don't you remember just before your operation that 'make 'em laugh' nurse told you that the average life expectancy*

after *a radical prostatectomy was 10 years. Now your operation was 4 years ago, so you're coming up to the half way mark. Let's see, another six years gets you around to 2014, so let's look on the bright side, at least you'll get to see the Olympics".*

Hope, *as usual sprang to my aid. "Why do people talk such hogwash about averages? Averages are absolute rubbish and I'll prove it". I waited for* **Hope** *to prove it.*

*"Now" he said in my mind "take a game of cricket, two batsmen go out to open the innings. The first one is out after 5 minutes and scores one run. The second batsman stays at the crease for 3 hours 55 minutes and scores 99 runs. Now, statistics would argue that the opening bats**men** stayed at the crease for an average of 2 hours, and scored an average of 50 runs each. Do catch my drift". I caught* **Hope's** *drift. "OK, now even if the average life expectancy after a radical prostatectomy **is** ten years, you have to allow that for all those who popped their clogs on the operating table and even more so, the numbers who were into their eighties and did so during the first couple of years or so for quite unrelated reasons. To arrive at an average there have got to be a whole host of people who are still around after twenty years or more.....you're sure to be one of those".*

Fear *wasn't slow in coming back with,*

*"that's all very well, **but,** you may be one of the ones who don't make the ten years...you've got to have a fair number of short-livers in order to counteract the longer-livers".*

I'd had enough, if the conversation was getting away from prostates and into livers, it was all getting beyond me, so I diverted my mind to an incident that had happened just before Ken and I decided to retire. A time when life was worry free, when the prospect of death was a million years away, and liver was just a nice thing to have with onions, bacon and mashed potatoes.

Chapter 16

A BOTTLE OF THE USUAL PLEASE

The Thatcher years were drawing to a close. We, in the property business had had a very good few years. The back-to-back deal was a wondrous thing to behold and Ken and I were lucky enough to pull off one or two of them before we decided to hang up our clogs. The last one *(which I don't intend to talk about)* had cost us very dearly due to the company we were selling to, going to the wall, and Ken and I getting stuck with the land in question as the property bubble burst, and the land we had purchased suddenly being worth half what we had paid for it. However, in reality, we should have learned our lesson during our penultimate deal, which, although it was, as Arthur Daly would have had it *"A Nice Little Earner"*, nearly caused a war between us, and one of the major companies we did business with. A major household name, but one that discretion demands that I do not name. In fairness, they were lovely people to deal with, and we had a happy relationship with them over several years. On this occasion we nearly let them down, simply because a good friend of ours decided that we were making too much profit and wanted to cobble together a little bit more for himself.

Let me explain. We had an Estate Agent friend...... yes its true; even estate agents had friends, who was going through a rather messy divorce. He had a beautiful house standing in several acres of gardens and paddocks. The Georgian house, beautiful as it was, was worth approximately one-third of what it was worth if you pulled it down and developed the gardens with an up market estate of des reses. Grant, for such I will call him, *(clearly not his real name)* was anxious to reach a fair settlement with his wife, and that fair settlement, in his mind, required him to sell the house at its, non-developable value, whilst reaping the rewards of its development potential at a later, but not too much later date. My partner Ken and I therefore agreed to purchase his house at its given value without planning potential, whilst entering into an agreement with him to use our best endeavors to obtain planning consent for its demolition and re-development *(never simply a done deal)* and thereafter give him a further sum which resulted in us getting a significant reward for our risk and effort, whilst he enjoyed a percentage of the overage. His divorce was settled. He divided the proceeds of the house sale with his ex-wife, and we proceeded to apply for planning permission. We were refused, but decided to take the risk of taking it to appeal. After two years, and many thousands of pounds in 'risked' fees, we won the appeal. In the meantime we had agreed, indeed contracted *(subject to planning permission)* to sell the land to our aforementioned friends at a certain price. On the day of the completion, Ken and I, Grant and his new girl-friend, and representatives of our buyers all sat in the ante room of the solicitor's office about to enact the completion which would, fill **our** wallets, do no harm to Grants, and leave our builder friends with a nice little development to get their teeth into. It would be improper of me to reveal the real sums involved, BUT in order that the principles can be fully appreciated, I will talk in purely illustrative terms

Let us suppose that we had a contract with Grant (let us call him **Mr. A**) to BUY his land for £100,000. In turn we (let us call us **Company B**) had entered into a contract to SELL the land, once completion had taken place to our end buyer (let us call them **Company C**) for £200,000. The magic about back to back deals in the olden golden days of less than 1990, was that *the middle man* simply used the end purchaser's cash. The paperwork always had to be slightly fudged, but with good faith on all sides everything always went smoothly. **Mr. A** signs the land transfer and passes it to **Company B. Company B** passes to **Mr. A** £100,000 *(but only in theory because they haven't got it yet)*. **Company B** who now technically own the land (thanks to the transfer **Mr. A** has signed in **Company B's** favour), now signs a transfer in **Company C's** favour in return for reciving £200,000, of which sum £100,000 now passes to **Mr. A**. Jobs Oxo, and everybody walks into the *'Rose and Load's a Money'*, for a celebratory drink Everybody is happy, hugs and kisses all round, and we go on our merry way........BUT NOT THIS TIME.

We did the sitting around the table bit OK. The lawyer produced the land transfer, transferring the land to us for £100,000 to **Mr. A** for signature. Ken and I sat there with beaming countenances, beaming that was until Grant, aka **Mr. A** said.

"I want another £50,000 or I won't sign".

"You can't do that Grant, I spluttered, we have a contract"

"So sue me" said Grant…with a *grin,* because he was a *friendly* estate agent.

"Would you like us to leave the room" said **Company C** our friendly end purchaser, who could clearly see a battle of wits developing.

"Don't do that" said Grant our *friendly* estate agent…."I might just sign it *directly* in your favour for the same money that they *(meaning Ken and I)* are getting… £200,000". He looked at Ken and I…"sorry boys", he said, **there has been a leak"**. I looked at the floor; it looked dry enough to me. Then I got his drift.

"You are forgetting" I said, "that it's taken us 2 years, a lot of skilful negotiating, a significant sum in fees, and an expensive appeal to win this planning consent"

"That" said Grant, our *friendly* estate agent, with a smile, "is the way the cookie *sometimes* crumbles".

"We wouldn't do that to Ken and Basil" said **Company C** our end purchaser, bless their little cotton socks, as my mother always used to say.

"I see", said Grant, our *friendly* Estate Agent "honour among thieves eh"

"Honour - full stop" said the spokesman for **Company C**

Our lawyer….who was also a friend to us all, was looking decidedly uncomfortable.

"Would you like a separate room?" he said to Ken and I….to talk it over

"I won't leave Grant" (he's our *friendly* estate agent) "with our buyers" I said.

"We'll sit in the car" said **Company C** our end-buyers. And so it was. We went into our lawyer's private office. Grant (our *friendly* estate agent) stayed in the board room and **Company C,** our end-buyers went and sat in their car. I won't bore you with the deliberations….but; we did our sums and refused to budge. But so did Grant, our *friendly* estate agent. Eventually, after much haggling we agreed to give him an extra £30,000 instead of the extra £50,000 he wanted *(the breakthrough came when one of us mentioned the fact that his former wife might not be amused at what he had done).* Our end-buyers came in out of their car and the deal was done. We dispensed with the hugs and kisses, and Ken and I went for a consolatory drink in the *'Rose and What a Bastard'*

About a week later Grant (our *not so friendly* estate agent) called in our office full of bon homie. "Basil, Ken, thought I pop in a show that there are no hard feelings.... but be realistic, you were giving me £100,000 and making £100,000 yourselves. I didn't think that was fair, don't you agree",

"That" I said to our now *very friendly* estate agent "is the way the cookie *sometimes* crumbles" throwing his old line back at him.

"Look" he said "let me take the two of you to lunch, anywhere you like"

Well you can only harbour a grudge for so long, and certainly not when a free lunch is involved.

"You're on", I said, "Netherwell Place". Netherwell was a fine country house hotel about half a dozen miles from the office.

"It's a date", said Grant, our *overwhelmingly friendly* estate agent. "What about Friday?" Ken and I made a big show about consulting our diaries before saying "Friday will be fine" I said...Shall we say 12.30 at our office.

After Grant had left, Ken, who had a wonderful sense in fun in him, said, "look, let's go and have lunch there today and pave the way for a famously *friendly* lunch". So we did.

We were not unfamiliar with either the restaurant or the Maitre D', and having ordered a modest two courses at £12.50 per head lunch, Ken called Maurice the Maitre D' over.

"Maurice, what is the most expensive wine you have in your cellar?"

"Well Mr. J that would be a rather special Champagne, from The House Of Ruinart in Rheims"

"How much is that Maurice?"

"It is quite expensive Mr. J."

"Yes Maurice….How Much?"

"£695 a bottle"

"That sounds fine Maurice, now this is what I want you to do…………"

Friday was a pleasant day, Grant picked us up in his new Jaguar XJ6 *(courtesy of our financial injection into his pension plan)* and we sped off to the restaurant. Maurice greeted us effusively and gave us a table by the window together with the menus.

"Mr. J" he said, "will you be requiring the wine list?"

"No thank you" said Ken, he paused….."Just bring a bottle of the usual"

I have to say that first bottle of 'the usual' went down a treat. So much so that Grant, bless him, called to Maurice. "Another of the same, please Maurice" Ken and I nearly had a conscience, but we both managed to dredge up the willpower not to interfere in a discussion between a man and his Sommelier. I have to say that the second bottle tasted even sweeter than the first, *but* the sweetest moment of all was still to come. Grant called for the bill – quite rightly expecting 3 x £12.50 for lunch, and perhaps a further £50 or £60 for wine. – with the tip, a little under £100. He got the bill and opened it, and this is where Grant, our ***friendly*** estate agent showed his class. He looked at the bill which must have been pushing £1500, He looked up, he smiled, then he grinned, then he burst out laughing...he called Maurice over and gave him a credit card, and then still chuckling he looked at us both and said just two words.

"You Bastards". He paused before, still grinning outrageously he said

"But I am still £28,500 better off.

Ever after, Grant remained a close friend and a ***very friendly ... EX*** estate agent.

CHAPTER 17

IT'S ENOUGH TO MAKE YOU CRY-O

The wonderful Victorian orientated town of Tunbridge Wells *(well known as the home of DIGUSTED...OF)* had clearly not been informed of my impending visit.

The clinic of Professor John Hardly was prominently obvious, but unfortunately situated in a side road that wasn't. Parking was next to impossible, so I pulled up, next to impossible, and parked.

The door was discreet, with a brass plate and a brass bell push. After some deliberation, I read one and pushed the other. There was a discreet click as the door lock disengaged. I found myself in a pleasant but understated hall with a smart desk and an overstated receptionist looking at me with an expression of quiet competence

"You are Mr. Jay" she said.

"I know" I replied, relying on my irrepressible charm to win her over. Polly just raised her eyebrows to the heavens, as if to say...."Basil, can't you give it a rest for one minute?" I thought it was time to get normal. "I am here to see Professor Hardly" I continued

"I know" she said…..in a 'getting my own back' sort of a voice. "Please take a seat and I will tell him you're here" I resisted the temptation to fire back a smart alec response. Polly was, I am sure, relieved. I took a moment or two to survey my surroundings, they were, I think, the word is minimalist, but in a curious way that gave them a feeling of ultra efficiency.

Around the walls were various framed photographs of a man, (who I later discovered to be the Professor himself), with a pasted on grin, and a series wholly unrecognizable dignitaries. There were also framed newspaper articles about cryo surgery, and evidence of various awards being presented to the Professor.

"Professor Hardly will see you now" The voice cut across my trance-like concentration on the wall furnishings. "Please follow me" I followed her, Polly followed me, and if there had been a handy brass band I am sure that they would have followed all of us.

"Come in Mr. Jay, Mrs. Jay, sit down, can I get you a coffee? I hope you had a good Journey. Did you find a parking space OK?" every question was clearly rhetorical, because he followed without a pause with "I'm John Hardly, and I have a letter here from"…..he paused and scrutinised the piece of paper in his hand as if he had never seen it before…"from"….I expected him to say Basildon Bond, instead…"from Dr. Henry Draper….nice man" he went on, obviously hoping that Henry was not the unfortunate monika bestowed upon a daughter whom the parents had hoped would be a son. It was quite clear from his demeanor that he had absolutely no idea who Dr Henry Draper was.

"Let me tell you a little about cryo-surgery" he said. He then proceeded to tell us a little about cryo-surgery, but my concentration had welded itself to his opening sentence which I rolled around in my mind, quite shutting out his intense explanations. "Some say", he said, that cryo-surgery is in its experimental stages". Mental images of hamsters *(or were they guinea pigs)* floated in front of my eyes. I looked at Polly, she appeared to be far more attentive than I was, and so, I was sure that she would fill me in later.

The Prof. had stopped speaking and was looking at me expectedly. "Any questions?" he said

"No" I replied, guessing that he had just read off the same script that Dr Henry had used, hoping that he would not ask me any, and sure that, if there were any that needed asking, Polly would ask them.

"OK" said Professor Hardly "first I am going to give you an ultra scan.

Please pop up one the couch" why oh why oh why do nurses, doctors, and even professors expect people to *'pop'* everywhere. I popped up on the couch. He started to massage a small amount of jelly-like substance into my long lamented prostate region before carefully circling a round headed wand over the offending area. He angled the screen towards me so that I could watch the slightly colourful swirls that appeared to make up the area of the prostate bed. He gave me a running commentary which consisted of a very neutral explanation of what he was doing rather than what he was seeing. After about five minutes, he gave me a paper towel to wipe of the residue of jelly, said "OK Mr. Jay, you can get dressed now" and left me behind the screen and returned to his desk.

When I rejoined him, he came straight to the point. "It is" he said, "far too early for us to consider any form of cryo-treatment, so I will write to Dr Draper and tell him so.

He then went through a long and boring narrative of how a small group of notable doctors were working very hard on finding away to cure prostate cancer without surgery, about how many awards they had received, and about how high were their hopes for the future.

I did feel that this long (almost 10 minute) oration was a little unnecessary for my ears. It was not until I received his bill *(thankfully paid by my insurance company)* in the sum of…….. wait for it…….. sit down……. pour yourself a stiff drink…… OK……. Here it comes…… but before allowing you to jump to any conclusions, I need to tell you that I must have been with him for a full 26 minutes *(assuming you allow for the time it took me to park)* ……. And the bill was….£470. Equivalent to the thick end of a £1000 an hour. What did I do? I will tell you, I went straight to the library to see if there were any books entitled. HOW TO BECOME A PROFESSOR…..***QUICKLY***

But seriously, it reminded me of an incident from my youth… I was about 18 years old, still at college, but a Saturday boy at the firm to which I eventually became articled. It would have been about 1960. The firm was Jesse Holness and Company, founded in 1838. The son of the founder, though born in the 1870's would still, occasionally come into the office. A Chartered Auctioneer, well into his 90's. One Saturday Morning I found myself alone in the office with this wonderful old man, who shared the same name as his father 'Jesse'. His son, who was himself into his seventies, was Bertie and a character in his own right. But back to Jesse. Up until the particular Saturday morning I had hardly spoken a word to him. On this day, he tapped on the glazed partition that separated his office from the main office. I had already closed up, it being after one o'clock. I was just balancing the post book and doing other 'before going home' chores. He tapped the glazed partition harder. "Young Man, come in here, I want to talk to you". When you are under twenty and confronted by a man of over ninety, the name Methuselah comes to mind. "Sit down" he said. I did as I was bid. He said nothing for what seemed a long time, and then, apparently from nowhere he said. "Always remember, you can never smile through a typewriter". I was a little taken aback and assumed that his mind was wandering. He smiled. "Silly old bugger" he said "I bet that is exactly what you are thinking". That was in fact exactly what I was thinking. "Bertie" he said referring to his son, who was senior partner. "Bertie" he repeated, "has never been a people person" he paused and looked straight into my eyes. "You", he pointed his finger straight at me, "are a silly young bugger" his face was wreathed in smiles, and the tone of his voice showed that he was joking. "Were you offended by that?" he said,

"Not at all" I said, "it was obvious that you were joking with me and not serious"

"Exactly" he cooed. "But… if I had written you a letter and said 'you are a silly young bugger' you would have been deeply offended and written back to me telling me that I was 'A senile old fool' Within two shakes of a lambs tail, battle lines would have been drawn, and we would have been at war". He went quiet for a moment "you cannot smile through a typewriter" he mumbled "never forget that young man".

What, I can hear you say, has this got to do with Professor Hardly. The answer is nothing at all, but what Jesse Holness said to me next put everything into perspective.

"My old father" he said, "a long time ago, told me something else that has been of great use to me in my life, and will, I hope, serve you as well as it has served me" He stood up and walked over to a number of framed letters and photos on the wall behind him. "People" he said, can never understand that you pay for what a man *knows*...not necessarily for what he *does*". He handed me the picture frame which contained a bill dated sometime in the late 1800's. It was on Jesse Holness embossed paper and said, simply.

	£. s. d.
TO REPAIRING WELL	0. 0. 6
TO KNOWING HOW TO REPAIR WELL	0. 9. 6
TOTAL DUE	0. 10. 0

As I handed the framed bill back to him, he said. "Never forget, throughout your life you will pay people for what they *know*.... NOT for what they *do.*

Suddenly I saw Professor Hardly's fee in perspective.

Chapter 18

MAKE MINE A DOUBLE

My life was settling down. Professor H had made his prognosis. I had made one of the silliest mistakes of my life. Dr Alonso the man who had removed half of my lower lip with an apple corer, had not sent the result to my GP as promised, instead his secretary had phoned to say. "Mr. Jay"

"Yes"

"Dr Alonso has asked me to give you a call to tell you that you can pick up the result of your recent test any time after next Tuesday"

"Where?" I asked

"Just call at the hospital and ask for the result of your biopsy"

"The result hasn't been sent to my GP then?" I asked.

"Apparently not" said Dr A's girl Friday "I have just been asked to let you know that the result will be ready for collection after next Tuesday". So, in keeping with my uxorious rule of doing whatever a member of the fairer sex tells me to do, I presented myself at the reception desk of the hospital, and committed a blunder most embarrassing. The receptionist looked up with a bored and apple sour face.

"Hello" I said giving her a wide 'infectious' smile, and knowing it was 'wide' because it was making my ears twitch, and hoping it was infectious, because she clearly needed something to brighten her day.

"My name is Basil Jay" and I have come for the result of my autopsy" *(you will agree a simple mistake that any **idiot** could make)* Polly gave me a gentle nudge with her knee. The receptionist 'almost' smiled, she looked at Polly and they immediately went competitive with a 'Who can raise their eyebrows the highest whilst rolling their eyes to heaven at the same time', sort of competition. Polly won, but then she has been practicing for more than forty-five years.

"I think you are a little early" the receptionist said. I still had not got it.

"Oh", I answered, Dr Alonso's secretary said any time after Tuesday. She put me out of my misery.

"Considering you are standing in front of me" she said, "you are a tad early for the results of your **AUT**-opsy, I would guess that you must have come for the result of your **BI**-opsy" She emphasized the **BI**, and suddenly, Being naturally bright, I got it. Luckily I don't embarrass easily, and with a well travelled, man of the world gesture, I said expansively…. "Whatever". She gave me an envelope. It had my name on it. So I opened it. Well you would, wouldn't you? It was a copy of a letter Dr Alonso had written to the lovely Nita and read. *"I have examined this chap, and took a small sample for analysis". There is no sign of malignant tissue, and I would say that his lips are sunburned…. Probably caused by staying out in the sun too long without suitable screening"* Wow! dead clever these medico's. However, as I thought it was possible that he was giving me the all clear, I felt it was appropriate that Polly and I should make an evening of it at our local hostelry, an inn , by name, The Dog and Bear, with a history which goes back as long as your arm *(how ever long that might be)*. The fare is delicious, and the wine excellent. However, I kid you not, there is one item on the menu that I have never dared try, nor indeed even enquired about… it is their renowned DOG AND BEAR BURGER. It makes a change from beef and cheese I suppose.

Life now settled down at a regular pace where winter followed summer which followed winter which… etc etc. There had been one addition to my medication. Well, not so much an addition as an alteration. My Hormone therapy was no longer six months on and six months off, it was now continuous. It was this alteration that put me under the knife again. I had re-started my oestrogen intake full time on or about August 1st 2008, and everything appeared to be going according to plan. Although it must be said that my hot flushes were a match for any of the other girls and my jumpers were gradually acquiring that 'sticky out' look again. I carried a fan, ignored the men, and closeted myself in dark corners with the other girls talking about grandchildren, a beautiful little top for just 20 Euros, and the best way to make rice pudding without it going lumpy.

And then, one morning I noticed that the source of my newly acquired 'sticky out' jumper, was no longer soft and pliable, but, particularly on the right, surrounding a hard, squash ball sized, lump.

"Polly" I enquired in measured tones, measured, that is, against a Richter scale of about 23.4 "I appear to have acquired a lump"

"Where?" she said, ever practical

"Well" I replied, "to give you a clue, from the front, I am in danger of looking like Quasimodo from the back"

"Let me have a look" she said. I let her have a look.

"Well", she said, "obviously a side affect of the hormone treatment."

"Surely more of a 'Front Effect" I replied, "I now look like a lop-sided Dolly Parton".

"Why don't you make an appointment to see Karen?" she said

"I think I jolly well will" I replied…always happy to go and be investigated by comely lady doctors. Karen *(no relation to the diabetic specialist in Kent)* was such a Lady Doctor who had left her Lancashire home to set up in, and administer to, the ex-pat residents of Los Cristianos in Tenerife. With an incredibly clever play on words, I always referred to her as 'The Lancashire Lass'. I picked up the phone and wandered out on to the terrace,

"Can I speak to Karen Please?"

"That's Basil, isn't it" the voice was that of Julie, Karen's receptionist, and someone who I knew well enough from my many visits, mainly for blood tests and scans, that she recognized my voice.

"Hello Julie" I said, "any chance of a quickie - word" I hastened to add in case she got the wrong idea.

"'Fraid not Basil, at least, not just at this moment, Karen is very busy with surgery and falling a bit behind. "Can I Help?"

"I am sure you can" I said, I have a small problem and wondered if Karen could fit me in tomorrow for ten minutes?"

I'm sorry Basil, but we are absolutely choc-a-bloc. Friday 10.15 is the absolute earliest I can manage".

"OK Julie", I said, "that'll be fine. Can you put me in for then?"

"Consider it done" she said. So I considered it done.

"see you Friday". I said I came in from the terrace.

"Karen is very busy" I told Polly, "she can't see me until Friday"

"Popular lady" replied Polly.

"She's popular because she has lots of *Patience* I said, and she has lots of **Patients** because she has lots of **Patience.**" I laughed at my rather clever joke.

"Eat your cornflakes" said Polly.

I got up very early on Friday ready to discuss the latest in medical breakthroughs with 'The Lancashire Lass'.

"Good Morning Julie" I said, "I'm early"

"Good Morning Basil" she said, "you're late". I looked at my watch, discreetly. She looked at the clock on the wall, pointedly.

"It's only 10.25" I said

"It's now 10.25" she said. At least we were agreeing on something.

"I'm five minutes early" I said.

"You're ten minutes late" she said.

10.30" I said

"10.15" she said

"Oh" I said "Sorry"

"No problema" she said. "Just take a seat and Karen will try to see you before lunch".

"I grimaced"

"She laughed"

"Sit down" she said, and Karen will fit you in as soon as she can"

I sat down, and Karen fitted me in as soon as she could.

"Morning Basil" said Karen as I eventually walked through her door. "How are you?"

"I've got lumpy humpty dumps" I whispered, in case the walls were listening.

"You're on Bicaltumacide, are you not?" she said, as a

doctor being well in-doctrinated into my medical history, but non-the-less looking at her computer screen.

"Am I?" said.

"That's what your records tell me" she said.

"If that's oestrogen" I smiled knowingly, "then I'm your girl"

"You're my girl" said Karen "It will be a re-action", she said, "boy and girl hormones don't mix"

"I realize that now I said, 'boy hormones' want you to enjoy romantic interludes deeply and often, while 'girl hormones' just give you a headache.

I was disappointed she didn't tell me that it was a 'side effect' because I was looking forward to testing the side effect - front effect joke that had fallen so flat on Polly, a Kentish Gal, on Karen, a Lancashire Lass. "Take your blouse off" she said with a broad grin….I took my blouse off with a fluttering of the eyelashes. She prodded and probed, serious now. "Almost certainly nothing to worry about she said, but we better be on the safe side…I am going to send you for a mammogram. You can either go to the Green Hospital"

"Or the Adeje Clinic" I finished for her, having been down that route a couple of times before for scanned photo's of other parts of my anatomy.

"If you're going to Adeje" she said, reading my mind, "just after lunch is usually the quietest time." She stood there awaiting one of my quick, but tasteless ripostes.

"Can I put my shirt back on" I asked. I had lost the taste for jokes.

I left the surgery and walked down to the promenade in front of the Gran Arona Hotel. *(no, I haven't missed the 'D' off, it's Spanish)* I sat on a bench and looked at the boats scudding across the millpond like sea. "Sod It" I said to myself, "Not again".

I drove back towards the golf, phoning Polly to suggest she met me in the Golf Club car park. Polly was there when I arrived. It was barely 12 o'clock, but an early lunch was clearly called for. As we were planning to go to Adeje at about 2 o'clock, we decided to have lunch at our favourite lunch time retreat, The Camel Park, our name for the lovely El Cerro de Luna (The Hill of the Moon) an absolute oasis of calm and tranquility, with each table set in solitary, palm tree secluded, splendour. We ate tapas, and sipped our way through a bottle of Vina Sol, the delightfully light local wine from the north of the island. We passed on the pud, but soon Polly had made short work of a local Baraquito, and I had drained my café con leche - con chupito till both the cup and the glass were way beyond empty. With no further excuse to stay, we went. Next stop Adeje.

Polly parked the car whilst I presented myself at reception.

"Hello" I said to the pretty, though buxom, receptionist. "I have an appointment for a scan" I showed her the card that Karen had written out for me. She looked at me blankly, I tried again. *"Hola, tengo un appointamente con el medico para un….um….um….um…**scano**"* (the last word spoken, more loudly, because, as every Englishman knows, if you speak **very** loudly to a foreigner, - in fact pretending they are deaf helps, it makes it easier for them to understand. Her mouth turned up at the corners and she pointed to a door in the corner through which she clearly wanted me to walk. A gift of languages is a wonderful thing, and I have been surely blessed. Through the door was another desk with a very severe looking lady who glared at me. She had a sign on her desk which read INTERPRETER. So much for **my** Spanish.

I eventually made, my mission clear, but only by speaking in English, at which time the interpreter told me to take a seat. I took a seat. Long before my buttocks had melded to the uncomfortable contours of hospital plastic, a nurse appeared with a smile. *"Hola"* she said, *"Señor A Add Es"*

"Si" I responded, *"pero en ingles decimos EEE DES"*

"Vale", she said…"Please come this way Mr. EEE DES". She smiled, I chuckled, and all was well with the world.

You all know how scans work so I won't bore you with a blow by blow account. After it was over however, I was surprised to be told that if I took a seat in the waiting room, I could have both the scan and a written report in just a minute. I sat in the waiting room, I waited, and was pleasantly surprised to find that she was only 59 minutes adrift with her time assessment because, the big hand had crept around the clock-face only once before I was presented with the scan, and a written report. But I was not complaining because as I read the report I realized that 100 hours plus of Spanish lessons had hardly touched upon the medical vernacular. Next stop was to the 'Lancashire Lass' again.

Karen read the report carefully before telling me that what had developed was a form of Gynecomastia *(popularly referred to as Moobs),* but mine were caused, not by some re-action to twelve Mars Bars before breakfast, but by my current intake of oestrogen. She stressed that it was quite benign, and nothing to worry about, beyond the extreme discomfort that she was sure I would be feeling….bless her. Her parting suggestion was that I 'popped in' to see my GP when I got back to the UK.

It was May 2009 before I had the opportunity to do any 'Popping', but, on May 19th I did 'Pop' in to see the lovely Nita, by which time the lump on the right hand side had grown rather larger, but there was by now a lump on the left hand side trying desperately to catch up. Let's cut to the chase….an appointment was made for me to see a certain Lady Surgeon, Her name was Sue Brown, and she hung out at my second home Winterlands Private Hospital where I had been an overnight house guest on a number of occasions, and a day visitor many more. She prodded me, she probed me, she ultra-sounded my lumps, and finally advised me that, whilst duly cognizant of the Tenerife scan results, which she agreed suggested the lumps were benign, she felt duty bound to recommend a further scan, almost certainly to be followed by a double lumpectomy. That was her recommendation. By this time the discomfort was considerable, and I was also concerned about attracting the unwelcome attentions of 'a certain kind of man' so I agreed. I had the scan the following day, and thereafter the process was pretty quick and within a couple of weeks I found myself back in Winterlands, discussing babies and fashion designs with a procession of nurses who clearly wanted to make the acquaintance of 'double lumpectomy man'.

The night before the operation, possibly encouraged by a recent evening of jokes at the golf club, I had a curious dream.

I was on the first tee on the links course on Golf Del Sur, a place from where I have topped, sliced and hooked many a memorable drive. But, also a place where for a particular monthly golf tournament, an open-sided marquee is erected to provide 'half-way' house refreshments. However, on this occasion there were no tapas laden tables. There were no admiring gallery; there were no smiling golf club staff. There was simply the 'Lancashire Lass' and 'The lovely Nita', attended by Dr Henry Draper, Mr. Breading, Surgeon Sue, the Po faced interpreter from Adeje, and the car park attendant from Book One of this trilogy. I was lying on a couch whilst golfers were asking for permission to 'Play Through'. The 'Lancashire Lass' came up to the couch upon which I lay, she had a beautiful Black Cat on a lead. The cat jumped up on my feet, and then walked right across me until it reached my head, where it stopped and purred before it jumped off the couch, raised its tail to show a single eye, and stalked off into the distance. Before I could recover, in came the 'Lovely Nita' leading a beautiful Golden Labrador, who sniffed my feet, cocked his leg against the foot of the couch, walked up to my head-end, sat down and gave a few woofs and a short howl, and then walked off dragging the 'Lovely Nita' with him. At this stage, Mr. Breading, the only man to ever hold my unprotected prostate in his hand, stood over me and beamed down. Suddenly they were all there, in a semi-circle around my bed. The golf course had vanished. The Tapas had gone. There was no-one asking to play through, Just Mr. Breading, Dr. Harry Draper, Surgeon Sue Brown, The po-faced interpreter, the sullen car park attendant from book one, the Lancashire Lass and the lovely Nita, all looked down on me with fixed and supercilious grins. Mr. Breading, the only man who…. (But we've done all that) boomed out. "Well Basil, we have given you an extensive CAT scan, and we have now had a complete LAB report. And, we are delighted to tell you. You are under the KNIFE again. The audience erupted into a cacophony of ragged, and quite unseemly chanting…BASIL… BASIL….BASIL….. I woke up, and there was my favourite nurse Sue with a hospital porter shaking me gently BASIL… BASIL… they are ready for you in theatre... Alec and I are here to take you down. In that moment, that magic moment halfway between 'asleep' and 'awake', it was not Sue, but Macho Man, standing there with a black cloth across his head, saying *"Take Him Down….. Take Him Down"*. Macho Man turned back into Nurse Sue, who…'took me down'. As she did so I recalled that only the day before one of my email joke suppliers *(thank you Mike)* – had sent me a joke about a black cat, a doctor and a golden Labrador. Well that one had certainly lodged in my subconscious.

I was wheeled in to the prep room, where I took the pre-med shot in the arm like the brave little soldier my mother has always told me I am. I pondered again about when, political correctness had required a nurse to say, "you will just feel a little *scratch*" which you didn't, instead of "you will feel a little *prick*" which you invariably did. And then I was gone.

I half-way came to in the recovery room some two or three minutes later, but was later informed by Polly, that about 3 hours had passed between them wheeling me out of my room, and wheeling me back again, attached, as I now appeared to be, me to various drips and drainage tubes connected to blood bags *(these I was soon to become very attached to as you will see)* and tucking me up in my hospital bed without so much as a story or a good night kiss. As it was only mid morning and Polly was there, I realized that I would probably have to wait for Alison, the night nurse, for that particular fantasy to be played out. This had been my fourth operation at Winterlands since 2004, and I knew most of the girls quite well. I had now had a bone in my foot removed and two more bones pinned together, I had had the anvil bone at the base of thumb removed I was treated as something as a celebrity when I explained that, as I have mentioned earlier, I had had ARF-rites so long that I was quite sure that, by now it must have become FULL-rites.

During the afternoon following the operation, Surgeon Sue came to see me for a chat. "If I had taken too much of the breast tissue away" she had said, "the nipple may have died, and we didn't want that…did we" I recalled my pre-op session with the make 'em laugh' nurse before my big operation in 2004, *(Book one, And The Tigers Come At Night)* then she had been spelling out the risk, albeit only one in one hundred, of not only my nipple dying, but the rest of me as well. Therefore on balance I thought a dead nipple was pretty much acceptable. However, Surgeon Sue had other ideas and she took great delight in telling me, with, of course, a broad smile, that she had left both nipples enough breast tissue to feed on, so they would keep their mushroom stalk capability for the foreseeable future. Sadly, such was not to be the case.

The operation had taken place before the end of May, I suffered a fair amount of pain over the following weeks, as the nipples, bless their cotton socks, tried to keep a tenacious hold on life. Sadly, not only were they losing ground, but the lumps once more began to form out of the remaining breast tissue. So it was that by the third week in July, I was back in Winterlands for operation number six in less than 5 years. On this occasion there was no thought given to giving the nipples emergency rations for the future, instead, Surgeon Sue intended to remove the whole of the breast tissue on each side. A double mastectomy, no less.

The operation was on Wednesday 23rd July 2009. I felt fine, although there appeared to be a lot of bleeding which resulted in my having two, less than fondly remembered, draining tubes, one on each side, leading to blood bags which the nurse measured and emptied regularly. On Friday 25th July on her rounds, I asked Surgeon Sue, what time I would be able to leave. She told me she wanted to see how things were over the week-end, and would have a better idea on Monday or Tuesday of the following week. I had to explain to her that that simply, was not possible, and that I had to leave that day, because Polly and I were attending our annual Swallow Reunion Golf Competition, which was commencing with a dinner on the following night (Saturday) with two rounds of golf on the Sunday and Monday. She laughed politely, thinking I had just made a very amusing joke. I waited for her to finish, and said.

"Really, I couldn't possibly miss it".

Gradually she began to realize that I was being serious, and sat on the edge of the bed so that she could be serious as well. "Look Basil, less than 48 hours ago you had a fairly serious and very invasive piece of surgery. Your whole body has got to get used to it. You have two drainage tubes inserted into the breasts, and they at the moment are discharging a significant amount of blood which has to be monitored regularly" She looked at me to see if I had understood. I put on my, 'Ah! now I understand' expression whilst saying,

"But surely I could carry those two little bags with me? I have watched the nurses empty and measure often enough, I am sure I could do it, and so could Polly – anyway, it will be quite a restful week-end and I wont be playing golf, just going around the course in a buggy with Polly" I looked at her to see if she had understood. She just held up her hands in submission.

"I cannot stop you discharging yourself, but I can, and do advise you that it will be a very unwise move" Knowing, as I did, far more about medicine and the healing powers of the human body that she did, I thanked her and said that I really valued her advise, but I would be fine. She stood up

"I want to see you on Tuesday afternoon at my clinic" she said… make sure you are there". She stood up and walked to the door before she turned and said. "And Basil, have a nice week-end, but don't you dare swing a club"

Our annual Swallows reunion was a long held tradition that I had started the previous year. As if we Swallows did not see enough of each other in our winter Tenerife home from October to April each year, I had thought in 2008 that it would be rather nice to meet up half way through the summer, for golf and good fellowship. The first re-union Polly and I had organized at the Forest Of Arden Championship Golf Course and Hotel. We had a splendid time and it appeared to catch the imagination as it was very well attended. I enjoy organizing such things, but in order to ensure that each year the emphasis would be different, and not decided simply on the price of a Kir Royale in the lounge bar, it was decided that the winners *(usually a husband and wife)* would, as well as receiving the trophy, be responsible for organizing the following year's competition. David and Cicely had been run-a-way winners at the Forest of Arden, for which they had received the new Basil Jay trophy of two penguins *(I couldn't find any swallows)* and the right, in the year 2009, to organize the event. And beautifully organized it was, at the splendid Hawkstone Park.

On Friday night Polly practiced emptying the blood bags with the huge elephant sized syringe, which sucked the blood out of each bag and measured it within the cylinder in gallons. She then had to enter the quantity on an appropriate form. I went to bed, with the tubes well attached within my humpty dumps, and the bags hanging on the side of the bed. I got through the night just fine, and Polly repeated the emptying procedure next morning. Before we set of for the Midlands *(The home of Hawkstone Park)* I experimented on what to do with the blood bags during my 'walking upright' moments. We discovered that if I passed the tubes inside a sports shirt, and I wore the shirt outside of my trousers, I could actually put the blood bags in my trouser pockets without them being obvious. And thus adorned, we set off for a week-end that we had been looking forward to since we left Tenerife for the English summer.

The journey was uneventful. We stopped for lunch on

the way, and arrived at the hotel about mid-afternoon. We did not see anyone at that time, but were advised that several of our group had arrived, and that a table had been booked for about twenty of us in the Hotel restaurant that night. I was feeling just a touch weary and so Polly suggested that a couple of hour's sleepy-byes would do me no harm. I had a couple of hour's sleepy-byes…. it did me no harm.

When I had awoken, one of us showered and shaved, the other just showered. We prepared to go down to dinner. I put on a pair of trousers, a loose fitting shirt, and my 'brave little soldier' face, and, first having emptied, and measured my blood bags, tucked them, one in each trouser pocket, and walked down to dinner stiff legged, as if I had had some sort of accident

The subject of both my operation and my bravery did not come up until I myself mentioned it, and that was not until several minutes after we had sat down. I jest, the subject did come up until towards the end of the meal, but only then because, when discussing 'Tee Times', I had to explain why I would not be swinging a club, but simply advising Polly *(wrongly usually)* which club she should swing.

The week-end went swimmingly. We golfed on Sunday, we gala dinnered on Sunday Night, we breakfasted before golf on Monday, and we lunched after golf, before everyone started their homeward journey. I went a little quiet over lunch, but managed to congratulate John and Sandra who had won the golf, quite convincingly, and, with the trophy, the right, to organize the re-union for 2010. We then said our goodbyes and walked down to the car. I was feeling more feeble with every step, and giving the car keys to Polly asked her if she would mind driving. Within a few minutes of setting of home I went from feeling somewhat feeble, to feeling definitely unwell, what started with Polly saying, "well you are seeing Surgeon Sue tomorrow" soon became "I am taking you back to the hospital right now". Sadly, 'right now' was a three hour car journey away, and it became one of the longest 3 hours I can ever remember. When eventually arrived back at Winterlands, I must have looked 'proper poorly' because with a minimum of discussion I was immediately admitted to the wonderfully dedicated care of 'my girls'. Surgeon Sue came to see me early next day on her morning rounds, I was feeling a little better, but presumably looking a little worse, because she did not once say

"There you are… I told you so",

In fact she said very little to me, but a lot more to the nurses. In the event, I was to remain in Winterlands for five days, and towards the end of my stay, Surgeon Sue, who explained that I had got an infection in the wounds, did take the opportunity to suggest that 'next time' *(did she mean I had grown two more humpty dumps that required removal)* I should take a little more notice of what the doctors told me. I decided there and then that, in future, I would take a little more notice of what the doctors told me.

I had my birthday, my sixty-seventh, in hospital, and although sent home again, had to attend the hospital three times a week to have the wounds drained and dressed. These visits certainly became great fun for our 'two special little people'. Our grandchildren Jack and Emma, seven years and five years old respectively, always spend a large slice of August with us, because their home city of Paris, where my daughter and her English husband have lived for more than 20 years, effectively closes for that entire month. Polly and I love August, and indulge the 'two special little people' by giving them a daily itinerary that they talk about for months afterwards. Howlets Zoo Park, Port Lympe, Lego Land, The Hop Farm, Leeds Castle, etc. etc. This year there was an additional attraction. I had twice been to see Surgeon Sue and had the draining, measuring, and re-dressing procedure carried out. During their first week with us, both Jack and Emma had sat in the car with Polly whilst I disappeared into the surgery for my administrations. Once back in the car they would bombard me with questions "Grandpappy, where do you keep going? Grandpappy what do your keep doing?, Grandpappy we want to come with you next time" Well, eventually I, who can refuse them nothing, gave in.

"Tomorrow morning" I said, "You can come with me and you can meet Surgeon Sue". And so it was. I went to reception with one little one on each arm and introduced them.

"Hello Frances" I said to Surgeon Sue's receptionist, "do you think Sue would mind if Jack and Emma came in with me?"

"Good Morning Jack" she said, "Good Morning Emma", and then to me "I'm sure she won't mind, but I will check". Surgeon Sue did not mind, and whilst I took off my shirt and sat on the couch, they sat on one single chair between them, the way that only little children can, and looked on with amazement at these two tubes coming out of my chest and terminating in two plastic bags half filled with either blood or tomato soup. Surgeon Sue, emptied and measured the bags, and then re-dressed the wounds. The little ones did not utter one word throughout the whole process. When she had finished, Surgeon Sue, turned to them and said….

"There, that's all done, you have been my first audience, but you can take you Grandpappy home now" She winked at me.

"Can we come tomorrow?" they said in unison.

"We will see" I said, and ushered them out of the door, saying my goodbye to Surgeon Sue, and shouting my goodbye to Frances, Jack and Emma, well they said nothing until we were back in the car, and then the WHY questions started. "Grandpappy, WHY have you got tubes in your chest?"

"Granpappy, what's in those two plastic bags?"

"Grandpappy, Why do you have to go and see that lady?"

and they were the precursors to a question and half-answer session that took place all the way home. My visits to Surgeon Sue became one of the highlights of that August visit, and I suspect eclipsed most of the *'other'* fun things we all did together.

By the end of August, except for two badly dented breasts, I was as right as rain again, and ready to prepare myself once more for the strenuous winter that lay ahead

Chapter 19

'FEAR', MUST NEVER WIN

Today is the 11th of October 2010. Tomorrow will be the SIXTH anniversary of the major invasive surgery which removed my prostate, my 'normal' romantic interludes, and for ten days until the 22nd of October, left me prostrate, *sin* prostate, and with an eighteen inch scar from pubic bone to belly button, and a similar length scar on the 'erotica remembered' section of my brain, to say nothing of a rather less than eighteen inch friend who would find it hard *(being, of course for the main part, the opposite)* to stand up for himself for many a long week, month…..and, well, just read on.

It was six years to the day that the 'make 'em laugh nurse', *(She whom I introduced in Book One)* oversaw, my pre-admission examination, and gave me so much grave news. You may recall, that this wonderful lady nurse, who, I have explained, clearly should have auditioned for 'The Comedians' gave me a pre-admission warning that **'One In A Hundred Men Don't Survive The Operation'** that was the **bad** news, But, if I happened to be one of the fortunate ninety-nine who **did** survive, *averages would suggest that -* the actual quote was '**On AVERAGE, most men survive**

TEN years following a Radical Prostatectomy', and **that** was the **good** news. No… it was more than good, it was **excellent** news. A pure nugget to file away, and pull out for scrutiny just several times a day for the next dozen (whoops! sorry) **ten** years. It would give me the chance to sub-consciously begin a count down…from 2004, to 2014, (or should, correctly, that be a count UP) Did I really care? I just knew what my Tigers would be telling me… 2005, ONE gone, NINE to go….2006, TWO gone….EIGHT to go…. 2013. NINE gone – don't make too many plans for next year Basil, you just might be a bit busy cramming for your finals.

You might remember from book one *(always assuming that you read it)* that my immediate response to part one of the *'make 'em laugh girl's'* prophesy had been to treat myself and Polly to 'a, *just possibly,* one- hundred- to- one', supper of the last request.

This was during my Kir Royale period. I had hoped that Kir Royales in sufficient numbers would keep the Tigers at Bay. They hadn't, but neither had old *'make 'em laughs'* **one in a hundred** observation proved fruitful. However, on this anniversary six years on I tried to keep that awful **'average life expectancy-ten years'** prognosis well and truly at bay. Sadly, in this *'information aware'* world' Mr. Google, bless him, is determined that anything we want to know is only one click of a button, by a questing finger, away.

I knew that, whilst, despite my fear of the daily dusted nugget, becoming, well, dusted daily, this six year old observation had stuck like glue to the darkest and most *inaccessible* corners of my mind, and although at the beginning, some days I would go almost five minutes without even thinking about, it, as time passed, for me in my waking state, it was philosophically filed away under Q, for *Que Sera, Sera.* What will be …….. will be. Sadly, not so with my Tigers who had fed on it, despite the fact that they had neither questing fingers, nor any sort of a relationship with Mr. Google.

I had moved on from my artistically exciting 'Kir Royale' period, and now enjoyed a slightly more mature, and less girly, 'Gin and Tonic for me', and a shared bottle of 'Dry White' with Polly, period. And, it must be said, that on this anniversary night, I allowed myself a slighter extended intake whilst wrestling with a *Lenguado A La Plancha,* at El Mirador in Los Abrigos. The reason was simple, on this special night, I needed to keep my Tigers quietly sedated, and unable to probe those dark and inaccessible corners previously referred to. Gin and Tonics in adequate quantities, I have found, make many such dark corners **totally** in-accessible – as indeed they make the location of your car keys, your car, the car park, and even your front door.

But on this anniversary night, my Tigers were not to be denied, and in that scary pre-dawn, I was aware of their sharpened claws digging into those same dark places of the mind where our worst nightmares lurk.

"You do know what today means, don't you" growled **'Fear'**

"SIX YEARS GONE…just FOUR to go". I heard, but I tried not to listen, 'Fear Will Not Win' had been my mantra over many sleepless pre-dawns in the years since Mr. Breading had played catch with my unprotected prostate. In the sleepless pre-dawns when either the 'demons of the mind' or a full bladder had teased me into wakefulness, to lie beneath the claws of that growling monster **'Fear'**, *I was proud of the many times I had told him to 'sod off', only to find that 'off' he had obediently 'sodded'.*

This night, was, however, a little different. An anniversary no less. A positive date for **'Fear'** *to dig his claws into. And dig* *he did. He had soon moved in to top gear. He started with a theme he had used before.*

"At least, you should see the London Olympics in 2012" he had growled, as if that was going to be the highlight of my 'how ever many' remaining years. "Let's see" he went on speaking in my mind "you were married in 1965. Your Fifty years is up, and Golden Wedding Bells will ring – Ding-a Ling-a-Ling-Ding in March 2015". He paused, as if pondering "But will they? Let's see, when was your operation now…Ah yes, October 2004, now, if we add ten on to 2004 we get 2014. Whoops, we may just have to settle for Ding-a-Ling-a-Boinnnnng". In my mind I could almost see him grinning. But he hadn't finished yet. "Moving on now", he began again, "what about 'The Little Ones', what about Jack and Emma. How old are they now, ah! yes, seven and five….oh, deary me" But I had had enough, it was time to remind myself, that 'Fear Will Not Win, Not Ever In This Life' and suddenly I knew just how to make him slink back into his place of dark pessimism…

I called for my very best Tiger friend, 'Hope', and 'Hope', never far away, leapt in to comfort me. He too started with his favourite theme.

"It's all rubbish this talk of averages" he purred, and then, clearly ,for my added peace of mind, felt the need to deliver a 'put down' to 'Fear', and build a place of sanctuary for me. "We need to really understand what 'average' means" he said, and, already I was getting bored. "We have talked about" 'Hope' continued, "the opening batsman scenario, let us examine this statement that seems to cause you so much distress" 'Hope', being a figment of my sometimes over active imagination, re-examined the statement both over- actively, and imaginatively "They have told you that the average life expectancy after a Radical Prostectomy is 'ten years'. I didn't need to be reminded of that statement so carefully stored it, well out of conscious thought's way. However, I felt something good

was about to happen. **'Hope'**, *after all, and not* **'Fear'**, *held the floor. I waited expectantly. Suddenly* **'Hope'** *was in full flow, and both I and* **'Fear'**, *gave him his head.*

"It is all about this word AVERAGE" **Hope** *said "There are three types of average. 'Mean', 'Mode', and 'Median'. Mean is the easy one, like our two opening batsmen. Add the two scores together, divide by two, and you have an average. Easy Peasy",* *there was a pause whilst* **'Hope'** *waited for us to both catch up. We both caught up. "Next there is the, 'Grouped Data' mode, this is where you cannot work out the 'Mean' exactly, because you don't know the values exactly.*

An example would be to work out the average height of 9 people, when you only know the exact height of the tallest and of the shortest. The best you can do in these circumstances is find, not so much an average, as a 'Mid Point'. Now, our ten year, 'kick the bucket' average undoubtedly falls within this 'Grouped Data' mode. Bear this in mind. Of each one hundred men who have the operation, **one,** *according to the averages, will 'cash in his chips' whilst still on the operating table. Another* **ten** *would probably have been in their eighties, and 'dropped off their perches' for a variety of other reasons, within a year or two. Another* **dozen** *probably drank themselves to the 'front door of the Grim Reaper' whilst, perhaps a further* **half dozen** *'met their maker' under the wheels of a number 8 bus, or a pile up on the M25.. OK, for this notional* **twenty four,** *their 'shuffling off this mortal coil' had nothing to do with their prostate operation or its aftermath, but they will still be included in the original* **'one hundred who lay upon that table'.** *Where, I ask you, is the average in that. And it does not end there. Of the remainder of our notional hundred, there were probably only two or three, who were, like you, in their early sixties, tall, good looking, literate, musical, a scratch golfer and super-fit"* (well they are my Tigers and they will say whatever I want them to) **'Hope'** *paused, but sadly not for long, he continued. "You catch* *my drift", I had caught his drift. He continued "You then have to consider the 'Moving Average' and then there is ' The Range', The 'Median Value', 'The 'Mode' which we all know is number in a set of numbers which occurs most So the modal value of 5634525 and 3 I 5. Because there are more 5's than any other num.."*

By now, out of pure boredom, his voice had trailed off into nothingness. I was gratefully back in the comfortable world of nod, and **'Fear'** had gone to some dark corner where he could stick his paws in his ears, and work out all the metaphors. Perhaps the Gin and Tonics had done their job after all. One thing I know, my last conscious thought was,....."'**Hope,**' bless him, has come up trumps again... I'm clearly good for another fifty years, and I obviously didn't need to take any more notice of BLOODY AVERAGES".

CHAPTER 20

THE BIRTHDAY

As I have said before, this book was always planned to be part two of a 'Trilogy'. A trilogy, the intention of which has always been to track the prostate path from its *very* beginning to its *very* end. An end perhaps where the final words spoken, by me, to Polly should be something memorable. Deep, but with far more meaning than *'Bugger Bognor'* (King Edward). *'Either this wallpaper goes or I do'* (Oscar Wilde), or even *'There, I told you I was ill'* (Spike Milligan). I think, perhaps something along the lines of.... *"Polly.... I have a secret bank account...its number is........its number...........umber is......Aaaaahhhhhhhh........."*

And so, it is time to bring this, book two, to a close, even though there is still much, which that, although already happened, is, as yet untold.

What I do wish to do is to visit, albeit briefly, two very special family events which were so important, and so enjoyed during the year 2010. Events which were a curious mix of happiness and sadness, but, which speak volumes about the closeness of families, and that emotive word 'courage'.

On May 16th 2010, my dear mother **Dorothy Ivy May** was ninety years old. Ninety going on seventy. She was born less than two years after the end of The Great War. A war in which both my paternal and maternal grandfathers fought and survived. She was a young auxiliary nurse during the second world war. It was through her nursing that she met my father, straight from the beaches of Dunkirk and to the commandeered country house in the Midlands which had been turned into one of the hundreds of large country house hospitals so desperately needed to accommodate the young men from those shell blasted beaches.

My father, John by name, and yet Jack to all who knew and loved him *(my daughter, bless her, named my beautiful grandson after him)* was just twenty-five years old. A regular soldier since 1933 when he was 18 years old. He had seen service in India and North Africa. He was a Staff Sergeant whose convoy of trucks was shelled almost at the end of its journey to the beaches of Dunkirk in 1940 Most of the men in that convoy had been killed. My father was horrifically injured. Injuries that were eventually to kill him - just short weeks after his 29th birthday in 1944.

My mother had nursed him during his long months in hospital. They were married on Trafalgar day in 1941. I was born in July 1942. Staff Sergeant John Alfred (Jack) Eades died on November 23rd 1944. My mother then joined the ranks of the thousands of young women, widowed and left to bring up their sons and daughters alone. She was just 24 years old. My mother never remarried. She devoted her life to me, as I now try to devote a very large part of my life to her. To involve her, as Polly and I always have in our own growing family.

I am sorry if that all sounds a little Maudling, but I need to paint the picture of the lady, who has spent her life alone, and yet I sincerely hope, not lonely.

She is without a doubt, the Matriarch of our, very large, family. She has never lost touch with my father's side of our family, and has always stayed so close to her own sisters, their children, and now their children's children. She is the one who, through, the more than sixty-five, years that have passed since my father's death, has kept the family together, with regular phone calls, with newsy letters. Never a forgotten birthday. Never a forgotten name.

We knew, Polly and I, that a bumper birthday to recognize ninety selfless years, was the order of the day. And bumper birthdays needed organization and a little bit of luck.

Bearing in mind that people would *(assuming they accepted our invitation),* be travelling from all points of England. The West Country, The Midlands, The North, plus a special deputation from Paris, and even representation from the USA. The choice of venue had, therefore to be, easily accessible. At the same time, the venue had to be close to mother's home in Eastbourne. We chose The Powdermill Hotel, at Battle in East Sussex. A beautiful country-house hotel from where could be seen Senlac Hill, the actual site of the Battle of Hastings in 1066.

Next was the guest list. This spanned an unbelievable FIVE generations. From Auntie Rita, my father's sister, albeit only a few years my senior, to the children of the children of my mothers nieces *(on each side).*

The invites went out, and the venue was booked, A car was ordered to collect mother and deliver her to Powdermill *(an arrangement that we later changed)* and all systems were go.

And then three bombshells. The first, the most awful of all. Tommy Spark, the husband of mum's eldest sister's daughter Betty, was taken ill, and removed to hospital, where, tragically and unexpectedly, on April 11ᵗʰ, he died. I will talk more about Tommy in another connection, in the next chapter, but it was news that really rocked us on our heels. Nothing was said, but we guessed that none of Tommy's immediate family would feel the least bit like celebrating a birthday, less than a month after the funeral of a man who was such a pivotal part of the lives of our northern cousins. But we reckoned without the deep and genuine feelings everyone held for mum. I had, of course, written to Betty, my cousin and Tommy's wife, with our deep, deep sympathy, and I received back a beautiful letter, which apart from talking about Tommy, told me that the whole family were looking forward to joining us on May 16ᵗʰ, because everyone wanted to be there to share that special day.

The second bombshell, obviously not so tragic, was the news, shortly before the birthday lunch, that Mum's youngest and closest sister *(closest, demonstrated by the fact that they phone each other twice a day, never less, than one chatty hour each time – the first to check that they have both got up, and the second to tell each other to go to bed)*. Her name is Gwen, she is, without doubt, the joker of the family. The news was that Gwen had been taken into hospital, and, whilst not in a critical condition, would not be able to travel to Eastbourne for the birthday lunch.

And then, the third. We had a flight booked out of Tenerife, our winter home, for the 11ᵗʰ May. This gave us a few days to make sure everything was in place, and to entertain 'Bunty' *(Margaret if you read the birth certificate)* the daughter of mum's second sister Lou, who was flying in from Seattle in America, and whose plane was due to land at Heathrow, just two hours before ours landed at Gatwick on May 11th. This gave her adequate time to transfer from airport to airport, whereupon we would take her back to our home in Lenham, where she would enjoy a few quiet days with us before surprising Mum at the Powdermill. WROOOOOOONG. In Iceland, the fates were throwing the runes. Let us, the runes had said, send a billion trillion trillion tons of volcanic ash up into the far blue yonder, so that we can stop ALL international flights, and so ensure that Basil and Polly cannot get back for his mother's birthday. The fates, jolly nearly succeeded, but, they reckoned without the power of love. Tim, our eldest son collected Bunty from Gatwick *(Her plane had not been cancelled, but had presumably been re-routed over somewhere like Wigan, whose air space the volcanic ash would not have dared to invade)* and moved into our house to keep her company whilst awaiting our arrival. Jeremy , our youngest son liaised with Powdermill to make sure every last request had been looked after. The man upstairs must have stuck his fingers in the volcano, because, on the 14th May, just one full day before the event, flights were once more available from Tenerife to Gatwick. And so it was we enjoyed the best of all worlds… we were there on time, and our children had done all the work.

There is not much more to say about a luncheon that went like a dream. We had cancelled the car, and I had myself driven to Eastbourne *(dropping of Polly at Powdermills en route, so that she could make sure that everything was in readiness)* and I had driven on to collect mum, who, I have to say, we had told we were taking to our regular 'One Sunday each Month' restaurant 'The Mirabelle', tucked quietly away in the Grand Hotel in Eastbourne, for a Birthday Lunch. I had told her that, providing the boys were not too busy, they were going to try and join us. I'm sure she was a little unhappy that we would let such a landmark birthday pass with such scant recognition, and I suspect that she was a tad put out when I arrived on my own….I explained that Polly had been a bit busy and would join us at the restaurant later. We set off, and Mum soon said, "this is not the way to the Mirabelle" *(never underestimate a ninety year old)*.

"Well no" I said, "as we go there every month, I thought somewhere different would be nice"

"Where are we going?" She asked, The Powdermill in Battle" I said

"Isn't that the place that you and Ken *(my business partner of long ago)* tried to buy in the eighties?" she said. Hold on, this lady is ninety years old, she's not supposed to remember things like that,

"Well" I said, "yes, we were interested, but we were out-bid"

"Probably just as well" she answered. There was a longish pause, "Do you know, she said, it's my birthday and I have had no card from Betty…she doesn't usually forget, but of course, with poor Tommy, she probably has a lot on her mind"

"She must have" I said.

"And Kelly" (Betty's Grand-daughter) she never ever forgets….but she seems to have this year". She was quiet for several minutes. "They have an excuse", she said, "but do you know, I haven't heard from Rita?" (Dad's sister) "nor Jill and the family" (Dad's sister's children). "Perhaps they are all busy"

"Perhaps they are" I said, as we thankfully reached, and turned into, the long meandering drive of The Powdermill Hotel.

"Oh Bless him" said mum, "there's Tim waiting for us". It was true, Tim was on sentry duty, and the minute he saw us turn into the driveway he ducked inside to warn the waiting guests.

"I'm so glad Tim is here" said mum, "do you think Jeremy managed to get here as well?"

"I hope so", I said. "I am sure he will have done his best. We parked, Tim rushed out to open the door for his Granny, we walked into the Hotel Lobby where, not only Polly and Jeremy were waiting, but also Tania, Nigel and Jack and Emma… all the way from Paris.

"Happy Birthday Auntie Nan" the little ones shouted *(they had never quite grasped the concept of a GREAT Granny, and had called her Auntie Nan since they were old enough to talk)* Everybody hugged, Granny started to walk towards the restaurant.

"Silly Auntie Nan" said Jack…"we are in here". He took her hand and led her towards the door of the private room we had booked. He opened the door. I moved up to take Mum's arm, She walked into the room and simply could not take it in as a roomful of people all shouted HAPPY BIRTHDAY'

"Oh Barry" she said ". There's Betty" she looked around…. And Bunty, she's in America, what is she doing here? "

"Mum" I said, hugging her close "they are all here for your birthday". She looked around, speaking their names out loud.

"Rita, Jill, Linda, Alan" she took a step further into the room. "Michael, Sue… and there's Kelly and Kevin and their little ones," The roll call went on, "Tony and Brie, ."She was looking from side to side, There's Paul and Pippa with Freya and Tilly", And so it went on. I took her to a table laden with cards, flowers and presents. "I wonder", I said, holding both her hands in mine, "if this is why the postman hasn't been delivering this week?"

Mum moved from table to table hugging, and chatting to everybody there. We all took a wealth of photos. In that special room of family, the ages ranged from just one year old, to a very special ninety years old

The rest of the lunch went in a slow motion dream. But the *'magic'* had all happened in those first, precious, moments

CHAPTER 21

THE WEDDING

I have mentioned Betty, the daughter of Mum's eldest sister, and about the very sad death of Tommy, her husband, and father of Michael, Diane and Pippa. This led to, what for me was a particularly poignant event. The wedding of Pippa, to Paul. I played a central role in that wedding, a role that really started over forty years ago.

I don't remember quite when I first met Tommy Spark. I must have been about ten, and living in the village in which most of my mother's family had lived for a great many years. The village was Whittington, a small hamlet in those days with just two or three buses a week into the county town, of Lichfield, the city dubbed the 'Mother of the Midlands' and the much revered home of Dr. Samuel Johnson.

I had a cousin, Betty. She was a few years older than me, and was very very pretty, particularly in the eyes of a ten year old cousin. One day she came to see Granny Goulding, *(my mother's mother)* with whom I was living, to introduce her new boy friend – Tommy. Wow! was I impressed. Tommy was not a tall man, but he looked absolutely splendid in his Army uniform. He had a smile that you could see from the other end of the village, and a sense of fun that radiated to all about him. Tommy was in the army…that was a plus from my point of view, but then a double plus… Tommy was a bandsboy, and he played in the Regimental Band. More than that….he was at Kneller Hall School of Music. To my young sensibilities, it was no wonder that Betty wanted to go out with him.

Tommy and Betty were married in 1952, and for much of the next twenty years travelled the world together with their military family. After ten years as a bandsman, Tommy served in the regular army until the mid sixties, when he went to Scotland to teach music at the army boy's school. Where am I going with this you may be thinking. I'll tell you, because of a special event that happened on October 16th 2010, I wanted to share with you some memories of a man in whose place I was proud to stand on that remarkable day.

Tommy and Betty had two children Michael and Diane early in their marriage, and then had a rest until 1964 when Pippa came along. I would have been twenty two years old, and still used to see Tommy and Betty at fairly regular intervals. One day Tommy phoned me to ask if I would be Godfather to their new daughter. At twenty two, no challenge is too great, but it is only in later years than I have come to realize that being a godparent is far more than sending a card at Christmas and on Birthdays, And sadly I seldom remembered even that.

At my mothers birthday lunch I had talked to Pippa, along with all of the family. The sadness and grief was easy to see behind the smiles. Those awful first stages one goes through when desperately trying to come to terms with a loved one's death. Polly, whose mother and father had died within three months of each other in 1997, and myself, but, most of all my mother, knew the courage it takes to celebrate one person's happiness, whilst grieving for another. The whole family presence at that birthday lunch for my mother will never be forgotten.

It was some little time later that I received a letter from Pippa with an unusual, but wonderful request. She told me that she and Paul were to be married on October 16th, that the wedding had long been planned, and that they felt that Tommy would have wanted them to go ahead with it. Then the big question, would I, as her godfather, give her away. Of course, I did not have to think about my answer… it would be a great privilege, and an opportunity in a very small measure to make up for my unintentional failings as a godfather over so many years.

Inevitably, as the wedding approached I began to think more and more of what I was about to do. For just one day, I would be standing where Tommy should be, I would be carrying out, with great pride, but also sadness, a 'labour of love' which ranks amongst the proudest moments of any father's life. I remembered my own daughter's wedding exactly ten years earlier, the lump in the throat as I had walked her down the aisle, the pricking of the eyes as the vicar asked '*who giveth this woman*'. I knew that I would feel the same pride, and the same lump in the throat and pricking of the eyes. But there was more. I tried to imagine what Pippa would be feeling, smiling at me, but knowing that it should be Tommy standing there. Behind me would be Betty, Michael, and Diane, and their partners, and children. All with the same thought. Would, I wondered, we all get through such a day with our emotions intact.

The wedding was wonderful, the only glitch, and an amusing one in retrospect, was that Pippa was clearly intending not to fall into the trap of being 'a late arriving bride' at the church. She had packed her mother, and the bridesmaids off from the house with three quarters of an hour to spare. And then, 30 minutes before the wedding march was due to begin, she said to me "I think we better go now"…... and so we got into the wedding car and off we went. As we drove down the country lane to the church, we could see the Matron of Honour, sister Diane standing under the lyche gate gesticulating wildly. We drove all the way to the gate and I wound down the window.

"You're 25 minutes early" said Diane "go for a ride, there's no guests here yet". And so, for 20 minutes the driver meandered around the streets of Lemington Spa, whilst Pippa and I talked about, a million things, with ease, not once mentioning the Wedding or what lay ahead.

When we got back, the church was full. The service was lovely, everyone was very brave, but I knew we were all fighting hard to keep the tears at bay.

At the reception, Pippa, quite unbeknown to any of us, stood up and announced to all the guests. "I want to talk to you about my Dad". And then from the heart she told about times they had shared to together, about his humour, and about his never ending optimism. His love of partying, the way in imparted his 'can do' attitude to life to all of his children and grand children. His love of travel, and the example set by both himself and Betty of living a 'good life'

In a magic five minutes, Pippa brought Tommy, her father, into the room for us all, and somehow we all knew that Tommy had not missed the wedding after all.

Polly and I left the next day to go back to Tenerife. We had invited Pippa and Paul, and their two delightful daughters Freya and Tilly to join us for a holiday. We vacated our home to give them plenty of room and freedom, and moved into the identical villa of two close friends who were still in the UK *(an arrangement that is not uncommon amongst the Swallows of Tenerife)*. We live on a complex tailor made for children, and, as usual in Tenerife we enjoyed wall to wall sunshine for the whole time that they were there. During that week, I got to know Pippa, my goddaughter, very well, and although I would have given anything not to have taken Tommy's place on that day, I felt grateful that I had had the chance to perform an important and a significant role in her life.

CHAPTER 22

COURAGE

This book has been a great self-indulgence. It shows my usual 'cock-eyed' view of life, and would suggest I have no 'serious side', and, in the main, I would guess that is true. But, there is a corner of my make up which can, and quite often does, 'cry' with the best of them. It was important for me to relate the stories of The Birthday and The Wedding, because for me, these two special celebrations captured the real essence of courage.

You will now know that the two Tigers who try to pull me down, and then lift me back up again, are **'Fear'**, he of the deep growl, the growl that becomes a roar, and the sharp claws that are always trying to rip the meaning out of my life. Then, bless him, **Hope'**, he of the nuzzling calm, and the gentle purr, whose *logic* always shatters **'Fear's'** scaremongering, and sends him slinking back into the dark corners of my mind where he lies waiting, waiting for the next time, and knowing, always knowing that there *will* be a next time. I told in book one, of another Tiger who, in the early days, between the diagnosis of my cancer and the surgery, used to visit me. He was my philosophical friend,

I called him, **'Resignation'** but gradually realized that, it was not that I was simply resigned to my fate, it was not that I was simply going to sit in front of the television set, or on my Tenerife terrace with *a* good book (*as opposed to The Good Book*) and just wait for the man with the scythe. It was more a calm acceptance, not, of course, calm in those first worry and fury filled weeks, but an anger which became a calm acceptance once, as they say, the *die* was cast. I felt that I should have a Tiger called **Courage.** But I have to say that my Tigers *'Hope',* and *'Calm Acceptance'* are more appropriate. You see, I do not believe that it takes courage to accept the inevitability of life......and that is, of course, death. **The** Good Book, as opposed to simply **a** good book tells us that we have three score years and ten. Sadly, some have less. Joyfully, others have more. But whether more, or whether less, it is not in our gift to choose for ourselves. We all face an inevitable conclusion to our earthly journey, every man and woman who has ever walked this wonderful planet. Some of us are given hints along the way, as to the approaching inevitability. The commonest, but by no means the only, hint of all is the presence of cancer. And, having been given that hint, one fights it, because the human spirit will let you do naught else. But the fight in itself isn't courage, it is simply the *calm acceptance* of what will be....will be. *Que sera sera.* These are simple truths. 'Man with Scythe' may knock upon *my* door, this year, next year, five year hence, or when I am sitting in a old rocking chair waiting for my telegram from the Queen (*or hopefully even a future King*). But that is so of all of us, I no longer need to beat my breast in anguish, I will be forgiven my occasionally pre-dawn spats with my Tigers. But the expression, oft used, *'after a long and brave fight against his illness'* is a comfort to the people wherein the real courage lies, those who are left. And it is an important comfort. The fact, in my mind at least, is that *'calm acceptance'* does not mean giving up on life, what it does mean is simply to carry on your life as you have always lived it, laughing when you find things funny, crying when you find them sad; enjoying the company of friends, but more importantly allowing friends to enjoy your company. This brave *fight* that every one likes to think has been fought would imply, the raising of the fist to the sky, and with anger in your heart crying out *'why me?'* when surely the cry, should be a whisper, and the whisper should be simply, *'why not me!'*. I know, that through calm acceptance, and the right to indulge myself from time to time with pre-dawn lectures from my Tigers, quietly in my own bed, and privately in my own mind, I can enjoy the very privileged life that I have. But I do want to tell you about 'Courage'

On May 16th 2010 I was particularly reminded of the courage of my mother, who, at twenty-four years old, intentionally and determinedly set out on a road, not so much of loneliness, but of being alone. I think back to when I was twenty-four, a time of plenty, of fun and of freedom. I compare it with that which my mother endured at the same age, for her, a time of great grief, of aloneness, of austerity and of ration books. With no particular skills, she took life as it came, she faced up to every hurdle, protecting me, and giving me the sort of life that she could never have…That is courage.

I have some images firmly fixed in my mind. Some from my own vivid memories. Others relayed to me by close family members like my dear Aunt Rita, who was just 10 years old when my father died. After my father died, my mother was forced to give up our small flat in Wood Green, London. She moved in with my father's mother and his little sister Rita. Rita, and my mother shared a bedroom. A twenty-four year old, newly widowed young woman, and a ten year old little girl who had doted on her big brother. In very recent years Rita has become very close to Polly and I. We have sat on our terrace in Tenerife and she has told me how my mother would cry herself to sleep, night after night after night, in the weeks following the death of my father.

I remember, so vividly, a day in May 1949, I was 7 years old. My mother had applied for, and got, a job as live in housekeeper at a small private hotel in Margate. On that day, I remember us getting off the train at Margate station and walking towards Cliftonville, to an address at the top of a letter offering mum the position *'on a three month trial'*. We passed a wonderful stretch of golden sand, and I so remember my absolute joy. I had never been to the seaside before, and it was a wonderland. I looked at the sand, the colourful striped deckchairs, the donkeys with the small children, laughing and singing, riding upon their backs, the sea dotted with sailing boats with their bright white sails. A *real* wonderland, to a small boy from the grimy streets of a blitzed North London, still carrying the frightful scars of the terrible bombings of 1940.

I looked up at mum with my eyes shining bright. She was looking down at me... and for some reason she was crying. Seven years old, but I remember so well. She bent down and hugged me, and for many minutes we remained still, a tableaux, me not understanding, and mum, bless her sobbing into my hair. After a few moments, she stood up and wiped her eyes, took me firmly by the hand, and we marched briskly along the sea front, past the wonderful clock tower which celebrated Queen Victoria's Diamond Jubilee, and towards 'Dorian' a small private hotel overlooking the Margate Winter Gardens. A place that would become my home for the next fourteen years.

I have remembered that day all of my life. My joy at seeing the sea and the sand. And then my bewilderment at the tears and the hugs, and the sobbing. The visible re-assembling of the emotions, and then, the purposeful striding to the place that would become our new home. It was many years later that it began to make sense. That this was a young woman, still in her twenties, her young husband, my father, having embraced a lingering death from awful wounds of war, preparing to meet a new challenge, a new life, to be spent, by her choice, alone. A life, five years on hold, now about to begin again, amongst strangers.

On that Birthday Lunch, more than sixty-years later, I intended to, and tried to relate that story to a room full of close family guests, but even as I assembled the words in my head, I looked at my mother. Ninety years old, More than sixty-five of them spent alone. A lump came to my throat, and I could feel my eyes filling with tears, and I knew, in that moment, that it would be a story I would only ever be able to share through my writing.

It takes no courage to die. Courage is the act of living on when your world has fallen apart.

I think of that beautiful wedding, when as Godfather I stood in the place of a man who had been the centre of so many lives. I remember Pippa telling the room that she wanted to tell them about 'her Dad' And then as the Reception continued, of Pippa and Betty, Michael and Diane, celebrating an event of joy, raising their glasses to long life and happiness. Smiling at the anecdotes. Laughing at the jokes. As they had back at the Birthday lunch in May, when their wounds of grief were still new and raw. A whole family 'moving on',

It takes no courage to die. It takes great courage to carry on when your heart is breaking.

In Tenerife, this has been a sad year. I have seen three friends die. And I want through these pages, pay homage to three wonderful ladies, Pam, Heather, Celia, who have smiled through their tears, determined to be brave in front of friends, smiling when they don't want to smile, laughing when they don't want to laugh. I have talked about courage in the women of my family. I am not suggesting in any way that in that regard they are special. The human spirit is amazing, even as we all accept the inevitability of death. We all equally accept the inevitability that life must go on.

Wow…. The many friends who know we will be wondering if I have just employed a 'Ghost' writer, because what I have just written will not, to those who know me well, sound like me. But, as I have already suggested, this has been a very self-indulgent book. It has had its 'medical moments', but it has been more about some of the high, and indeed lowlights of my life. When I am not talking to my Tigers, I am happily convinced that I will live, if not forever, pretty close to it. When I do talk to my Tigers, I always now finish reflecting on a life that has had as many colours as a rainbow. A charmed life with no real tragedy. I wonder if I would have the same courage to continue my life 'business as usual', as I have seen in so many others.

So, how do I close this book of mixed emotions. A book where I have probably revealed more of my inner-self than is good for the soul, or certainly for the happy go lucky chap I have always been.

Perhaps a recent visit to 'The Lovely Nita' will put us all back on an even keel. As I write these closing words, it is Christmas Eve 2010, Polly's birthday. England has spent two weeks under a blanket of snow that has covered the landscape. A few days ago, in Paris, Polly and I had celebrated an early Christmas day with Tania, Nigel, and the 'Little Ones'. 2010 is the 'Alternate' year when Tania and family spend Christmas with Nigel's family. Our two days were filled with happiness. Jack is just three weeks away from his eighth birthday, and has reached the age in boys when hugs and kisses are not really the thing, but he shows his love in so many other ways. Emma is five. Emma has no such inhibition. Christmas dinner was over. Presents had been opened. Everyone was sprawled on chairs and couches, having eaten too much, drank just enough, and now content to watch the children at play. Emma comes and climbs on to my knee, she gives me a big kiss on the cheek, and then snuggles down with her head on my shoulder "I love you *so* much Grandpappy" she says. I can't speak, I just stroke her hair. Six words that make the world a wonderful place.

The next day we said our good-byes early, and drove on clear roads, but through fields of white, first northern France, and then, through the Kent countryside.

We go back to Tenerife for New Year. I have a consultation with Dr Harry Draper in February. He wants a blood test now, and the lovely Nita is going to oblige.

Basil Jay, please go to room 8. The display of the wall mounted computer has spoken…I go to room 8.

"Good Morning Basil"

"Good Morning Nita"

"How are you?"

"I feel very well, thank you". She locates my file on the computer.

"An easy day", she says, "just a simple blood test for PSA"

"That's all" I say.

"Roll your sleeve up, left arm" she says. I do as I am asked. She puts the tourniquet around my bicep and pulls tight. "Make a fist" she says. I do as I'm told. She puts in the needle and draws a syringe of blood. She sticks on a label and writes my name on it. "You're not well, are you Basil?" she says

"I'm fine" I say

"No you're not, we have been through a complete procedure without one single puerile joke" she retorts, "in my book that means you have something on your mind".

"It's not your book, it's my book" I say, and if you're not careful I won't give you a mention this time". I try to give a broad grin… it comes out as a rueful smile. She looks at her watch, but not in her usual agitated way. She picks up the phone on her desk and dials through to reception. "Is my next patient here yet?" she asks. She listens to the answer "good" she responds.

"Basil, we need to talk, the good thing about snow is we get a few 'no shows' so we have about ten minutes" she smiles…. "Now talk….tell me what's on your mind"

"It's been a strange six years", I say "until 2004 I had hardly ever been to the doctors, and certainly not to a hospital other than as a visitor, and now I have had two operations on my….."

"foot, and one on your hand", Nita takes over, she is reading off the computer screen. "A radical prostectomy, one lumpectomy followed by a full double mastectomy. Four bi-opsys including one on your lip. Add to that, six MRI scans, four full body scans, four weeks of radiation therapy. You have had ultra scans in Tunbridge Wells, and Mammograms in Tenerife. On top of all of that you have had a colonoscopy, numerous blood tests, a liver scan, and a tablet intake that would have pleased Moses, and, on top of all that the opportunity to form good working relationships with no less than four surgeons, three consultants, and numerous doctors.". She stopped and I continued.

"Don't forget the nurses" I said. She raised her eyebrows.

"Have I forgotten anything else?" she said.

"Of course Nita, I have even sampled the joys of being a middle-aged woman complete with 'hot flushes'" She looked at me with a pouty face.

"OK Basil, I know it's been a bit of a bumpy ride, but it's good to get these little things out of the way. The next twenty-five years will be a doddle."

I took a deep breath, and then, in my very best thespanic voice, one that would have had Shakespeare rushing to sign me up to read the soliloquy from Hamlet on opening night

"Nita" I said. *"**What the hell am I going to do** for **an encore?"***

Such was supposed to be the classic closing line of both my consultation with the lovely Nita, and indeed this book. But Nita obviously had other ideas.

"Ahhh Basil" she said quite determined that I would not have the last word. "I think I know what you are suffering from" She fixed me with a hard stare before saying "you are

clearly having a serious attack of *'self pity'*. Now then in the six odd years I have known you, I have recognized that you suffer from an overactive tongue, an over-developed imagination, an under-developed comedic quality that doesn't stop you trying. But, self pity has never seemed a problem, which, like stress, you have given much houseroom to."

She paused, before saying, "so go make like a pair of curtains."

"Que" I said trying to get back in on the action."

"And don't think you can get out of a little lecture by resorting to bad Spanish" She was in full flow. "Just pull yourself together"

"Ahh" I said, "hence the curtain reference – *muy listo*"

"It wasn't *very clever* at all" she said, showing a two word fluency, *(obviously gained on a week-end trip to Ibiza)*, that I never even dreamed she possessed. She carried on, but now her face was set in very serious mode.

"Did you tell me you did not see the inside of a hospital as a patient until you were 62?" I nodded. "Let me tell you something." I could never have guessed what was coming, and I would swear a little tear glistened in her eye as she continued. "Earlier today, I had to see, and not for the first time, a little boy just 8 years old. So far he has had 5 serious operations and I have never seen him without a smile on his face, poor little chap, although he doesn't know it, he will be in and out of hospital his whole life, and it's a life that is likely to end long before *he* is sixty two." She paused for breath, and I held mine, as I prepared for the continuing tongue lashing. It didn't happen. Instead she said quietly.

"*He* will never get to spend his winters in the Tenerife sun. *He* will never be well enough to play golf, or go for a swim, or spend lazy days over long lunches" she stopped again and I thought she had finished. Instead she stood up and walked to the door. "You are still one of my favourite patients she said, but I would like to suggest that you go home, take your wife out for slap-up meal, have a nice bottle of wine, stop feeling sorry for yourself, and **count your blessings.**"

I took me fifteen minutes to walk home, *(it's not far but I don't walk fast- particularly having been told off)*. I remembered another young doctor who had given me a lecture almost 35 years earlier. I had done exactly as he had told me. I reflected on the privileged life I lead. Long, *'swallow'*, winters in the Tenerife sun. Winters spent in the delightful company of now close *'swallow'* friends, friends met after retirement, friends with whom we have no baggage, friends with whom we have no *'growing up'* past, but enjoy a slowly *'winding down'* future in idyllic surroundings. Breakfast on a, usually sun-drenched, terrace overlooking the sixth fairway and the distant mountains. Golf in the sunshine whenever we choose to play. Long luncheons or dinners with happy people. I reflected on my close family English summers as a father and a grandpappy. A mother who has entered her **ninth** decade in robust good health. Two sons who live just a short drive away. A daughter, and two beautiful grand children who, although they live in Paris, are only two hours away, door to door thanks to the channel tunnel and Eurostar. I gave a passing thought to Macho Man, and a longer one to my bank manager friends of the 80's, and to my former business partner with whom I had enjoyed so many rib-tickling moments, not the least of which was with Grant the *friendly* estate agent. A full life, of wonderful experiences. I reached home and absent mindedly put my door key in the lock whilst ringing the doorbell. Polly opened the door with raised eyebrows (*a tremendous trick, because it enables you to keep you're hands in your pockets*).

"Where's the car?" she asked looking over my shoulder at a half empty driveway.

"I must have left it at the Doctors" I said vaguely.

"Let's," I said "walk through the village together and collect it, then drive to 'La Soufflé' and obey 'Doctors Orders' with an early meal." We sauntered through the beautiful medieval village that is our summer resting place, through the village square, lined with lime trees, standing like soldiers on parade. The very trees from which our Lime

Tree restaurant gets its name. We walked in comparative silence as I went over Nita's recent lecture in my mind. I decided that she had been right, a little self pity had probably crept into a place in my mind where there was no reason to give it room. And, if the truth be told, and I am about to tell it, I *do* count my blessings, every day of my life.

And I can't wait to tell my Tigers the next time they come calling without an invitation.

www.ingramcontent.com/pod-product-compliance
Lightning Source LLC
Chambersburg PA
CBHW030306290526
45785CB00001B/230